THE ANAESTHESIA VIVA

A Primary FRCA Companion

VOLUME 1

Physiology & Pharmacology

Second Edition

THE ANAESTHESIA VIVA

A Primary FRCA Companion

VOLUME 1
Physiology & Pharmacology

Second Edition

John Urquhart
Mark Blunt
Colin Pinnock

With contributions from Mark Dixon

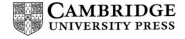

CAMBRIDGE
UNIVERSITY PRESS

CAMBRIDGE UNIVERSITY PRESS
Cambridge, New York, Melbourne, Madrid, Cape Town, Singapore, São Paulo

Cambridge University Press
The Edinburgh Building, Cambridge CB2 8RU, UK

Published in the United States of America by Cambridge University Press, New York

www.cambridge.org
Information on this title: www.cambridge.org/9780521688000

© Greenwich Medical Media Limited 2003

First published 2003
Reprinted by Cambridge University Press 2006 (twice)
Fourth printing 2007

Printed in the United Kingdom at the University Press, Cambridge

A catalogue record for this publication is available from the British Library

ISBN 978-0-521-68800-0 paperback

Foreword to the First Edition

The Royal College of Anaesthetists has revised its schedule for the FRCA examination from three parts to two, which, from 1996, will be called the Primary and the Final FRCA. The "new" primary examination syllabus includes basic anaesthesia and resuscitation, an OSCE, and has ten pages devoted to Anatomy, Physiology, Physics, Clinical Measurement and Basic Statistics. This formidable syllabus and the list of basic science subjects is in itself a daunting proposition for many prospective trainee anaesthetists. This book of Questions and Answers for the new primary FRCA examination provides an impressive catalogue of well-illustrated material for candidates contemplating the physiology and pharmacology parts of the examination. The book is equally relevant in the oral as well as the written part of this examination and is, based on an extensive experience of the authors in teaching candidates for the basic science parts of previous FRCA examinations. The authors have the advantage that they are clinicians teaching basic sciences and they have chosen topics from their experience of questions asked in the examination as well as topics that have particular clinician relevance. Many candidates for this part of the examination as well as their consultant teachers may see little clinical relevance of many parts of the basic science section of the syllabus for the new primary.

The present book provides in excellent preview of the range of knowledge presently expected by candidates for the new primary. It should riot be regarded as a substitute for traditional textbooks but it is an important supplement to such reading. It is certainly a very useful way to revise and particularly valuable for practising the *viva voce* part of the examination. Many candidates fail not because of lack of knowledge of the facts but because of lack of practice in oral question and answer sessions. Many senior colleagues would like to help their trainees with the oral part of the examination but they have forgotten the scope and detail of the basic science part of the examination and this book again provides a treasure chest of questions for the mock examiner. I look forward to further editions, which will include other parts of the new primary syllabus.

Professor Gareth Jones
Cambridge, 1996

CONTENTS

PHYSIOLOGY

1

QUESTIONS ON THE PHYSIOLOGY OF THE NERVOUS SYSTEM

1. COMPARE THE INNERVATION OF DIFFERENT TYPES OF MUSCLE

⊃ **This question involves the physiological differences between cardiac, smooth and skeletal muscle.**

Discussion will usually revolve around the different structure and function of the three muscle types focussing not only on the innervation but also the other comparative features. Skeletal muscle is uniquely striated, cardiac muscle acts as a functional syncitium and smooth muscle may be single or multi-unit. Comparative properties are shown below.

COMPARISION BETWEEN SKELETAL, CARDIAC AND SMOOTH MUSCLE			
	Skeletal muscle	**Cardiac muscle**	**Smooth muscle**
Structure			
Motor endplate	Present	None	None
Mitochondria	Few	Many	Few
Sarcomere	Present	Present	None
Sarcoplasmic reticulum	Extensively developed	Well developed	Poorly developed
Syncitium	None	Present	Present
Function			
Pacemaker	No	Yes (fast)	Yes (slow)
Response	All or none	All or none	Graded
Tetanic contraction	Yes	No	Yes

2. DESCRIBE THE CONTROL OF CEREBRAL BLOOD FLOW

⊃ The key to this subject is to understand the role of intracranial pressure (ICP) with regard to cerebral perfusion. The Monro-Kelly doctrine basically states that the contents of the skull are incompressible therfore any increase in one component will lead to a reciprocal decrese in the others. Normal ICP is 10–15 cmH₂O in the supine position. Cerebral Perfusion Pressure (CPP) is given by:

⊃ CPP = MAP – (ICP + JVP)   (where MAP = Mean Arterial Pressure)

Note:

- The brain weighs 1500 grams
- Normal cerebral blood flow is 750 ml/min
- Oxygen consumption ($\dot{V}O_2$) for cerebral tissue is 50 ml/ min (3.5 ml/100 g tissue)
- Grey matter receives twice as much blood flow as white (70:30 ml/100 g/min)

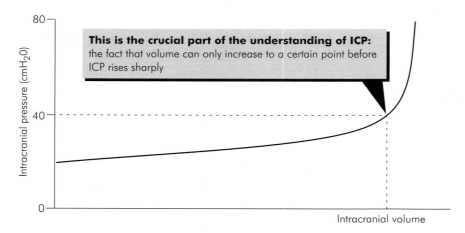

This is the crucial part of the understanding of ICP: the fact that volume can only increase to a certain point before ICP rises sharply

Autoregulation describes the ability of the brain to control its own blood supply. CBF autoregulates within certain limits. The cerebral arterioles constrict as the cerebral arterial pressure rises, protecting against too high a pressure, and dilate as the pressure diminishes, allowing more blood to perfuse the brain. This operates between MAP of 60–130 mmHg. Autoregulation is abolished by hypoxia, hypercapnia and trauma, and also to a degree by volatile anaesthetic agents.

3. WHAT IS THE MECHANISM OF THE KNEE JERK?

> ⊃ This concerns the basic reflex arc. Muscle spindle → dorsal horn →
> motor nerve.

The intrafusal fibre is the receptor component of the reflex and is embedded within the skeletal muscle fibre. It is innervated by Aγ fibres, which cause tightening of the fibre. The central sensory part is innervated by Aα fibres, which are fast, primary fibres to the cord, and by slower, β fibres to the cerebral cortex. The response to stretching a muscle may be static or dynamic.

Static response:
Receptor portion is stretched, a signal is transmitted for a prolonged period of time via the slow, β type fibres from the receptor portion.

Dynamic response:
This is the response to rate of change; a signal is transmitted only during the change in length, via fast, primary, Aα fibres.

If extrafusal fibre length becomes greater than intrafusal fibre length:
→ The receptor is stretched to accommodate this change in length.
→ There is an increased afferent signal

If intrafusal fibre length becomes greater than extrafusal fibre length:
→ The receptor is slack
→ There is a decreased afferent signal

Golgi tendon organs

- These lie in the tendon of a muscle at the tendon-muscle junction.
- The Golgi tendon organ responds to tension whereas the muscle spindle responds to length.
- The Golgi tendon organ sends inhibitory signals whereas the muscle spindle sends excitatory signals and probably have a protective function on the muscles to prevent damage from over stretching.

---

4. HOW IS MUSCLE TONE MAINTAINED?

> ⊃ This is achieved by summation, which is the adding together of
> individual muscle twitches to make strong and concerted movements.

There are two types of summation:
1. Multiple motor unit summation, which involves increasing the number of motor units contracting simultaneously.
2. Increasing the rapidity of contraction, which is known as wave summation.

---

5. COMPARE THE ACTION POTENTIALS OF NERVE AND MUSCLE

1. The resting potential is about -85 mV in muscles and in the large nucleated fibres that supply them. In a typical neurone the resting membrane potential is –70 mV swinging to +35 mV at the top of the spike,
2. The duration of the action potential in muscle is 5 ms-five times as long as that in the nerve.
3. The velocity of transmission in muscle is 5 m/s, this is $^1/_{18}$ the velocity of nerve transmission.

Expect to be asked to draw an action potential for a mixed nerve. An example is given below:

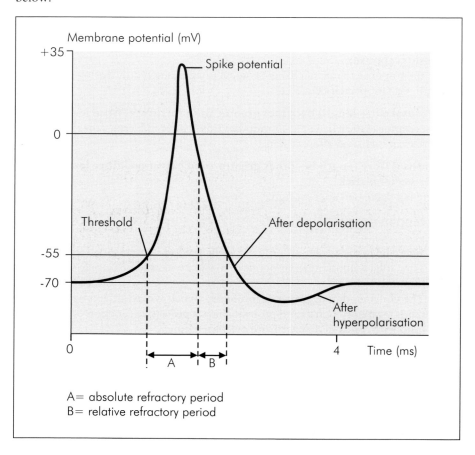

A= absolute refractory period
B= relative refractory period

The action potential in muscle travels longitudinally and then down the T-tubules which are extracellular becoming adjacent to the cisternae at the ends of the sarcoplasmic reticulum. The cisternae release Ca^{2+} ions, which interact with the troponin and cause contraction. A calcium pump then returns the Ca^{2+} to the sarcoplasmic reticulum.

6. HOW IS PAIN TRANSMITTED?

> ⊃ An overview may be useful.

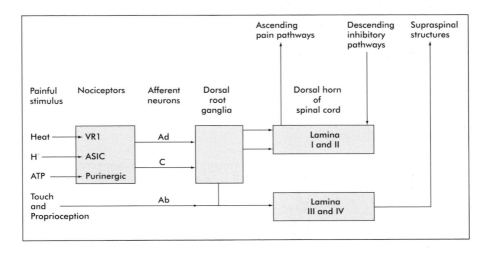

7. WHAT ARE THE FUNCTIONS OF THE VAGUS NERVE?

> ⊃ These are motor, sensory and secreto-motor. Point out that the vagus
> has three nuclei: Dorsal (mixed), Nucleus ambiguous (motor) and
> Nucleus of the tractus solitarius (sensory-taste).

Motor to:
- Larynx
- Bronchial muscles
- Alimentary tract (as far as the splenic flexure)
- Myocardium

Sensory to:
- Dura
- External auditory meatus
- Respiratory tract
- Alimentary tract (to ascending colon)
- Myocardium
- Epiglottis

Secretomotor:
- Bronchial mucus production
- Alimentary tract and adnexa

8. WHAT ARE THE FUNCTIONS OF THE EXTRAPYRAMIDAL SYSTEM?

⊃ **The extrapyramidal system: Regulates muscle tone, Governs stereotyped movements**

It consists of:

Subcortical nuclei
Caudate nucleus
Globus pallidus } – These are the basal ganglia.
Putamen
Brain stem nuclei

Rubrobulbar tract | These tracts accompany upper motor neurones
Reticulospinal tract | to influence lower motor neurone pathways.

Tectospinal tract | These adjust for eye and ear movement.
Vestibulospinal tract |

It is so called because it is **not** part of that system which forms the pyramid of the medulla.

---

9. WHAT IS THE BLOOD – BRAIN BARRIER?

⊃ **The blood–brain barrier (BBB) is formed by endothelial cells lining the cerebral capillaries and epithelial cells in the choroid plexus which are both sealed by tight junctions.**

Unlike a desmosome, the tight junction is circumferential. Thus, all transport must be transcellular.

Note:

■ The BBB is deficient in the region of the chemoreceptor trigger zone (CTZ)
■ Lipid- soluble drugs cross the BBB easily
■ The transport of amino acids and glucose is carrier mediated

---

10. WHAT IS THE RETICULAR ACTIVATING SYSTEM?

> ⊃ The reticular activating system (RAS) is a loosely arranged collection of fibres and cells in the brainstem.

1. The RAS receives and integrates information from all parts of the central nervous system (CNS).
2. The RAS outputs information to all parts of the CNS.
3. The RAS is responsible for arousal and RAS activity is implicated in the level of consciousness.

Definitions:

Forebrain   = Cerebrum + diencephalon
Diencephalon = Thalamus + hypothalamus
Brainstem   = Midbrain + pons + medulla

There are projections of the RAS to:
- Thalamus
- Cortex-directly

There is convergence onto the RAS from:
- Sensory tracts
- The trigeminal nerve
- The auditory nerve
- The olfactory nerve

11. WHAT NERVE FIBRES DO YOU RECOGNISE?

> ⊃ Normally this question will lead to a comparison of the role and size/speed of conduction in mammalian neurones (see table below):

CLASS	FUNCTION	SIZE (MM DIAMETER)	VELOCITY (M/SEC)
Aα	Somatic motor	12–20	70–120
Aβ	Touch, pressure, proprioception	5–12	30–70
Aγ	Spindle afferents	3–6	15–30
Aδ	Sharp pain, temperature	2–5	12–30
B	Preganglionic autonomic	<3	3–15
C	Dull pain	0.4–1.2	0.5–2.

Local anaesthetics block small fibres before large ones; pressure affects large fibres before small ones. This is why a motor palsy with preservation of sensation may be a consequence of pressure trauma.

12. DESCRIBE THE NEURONAL PATHWAYS THAT ARE INVOLVED IN THE INITIATION OF A VOLUNTARY MOVEMENT.

⊃ **Voluntary movement starts in the motor cortex (pre–central gyrus) but the thought behind that movement starts from the supplementary motor area or pre–motor area.**

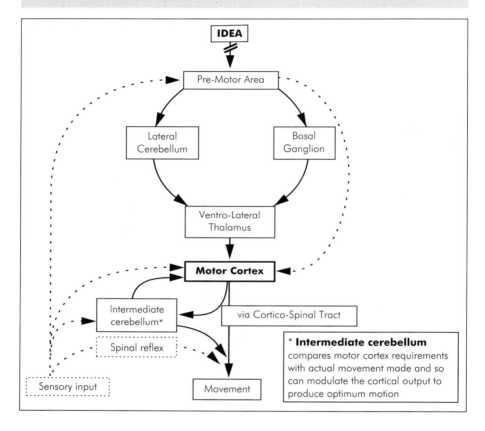

The impulse then descends through the internal capsule before decussating into the cortico-spinal tract to the anterior horn cell and then to the α motor neurone.

Within the corticospinal tract there is branching to help produce multiple innervation and so produce a controlled movement.

2

QUESTIONS IN CARDIOVASCULAR PHYSIOLOGY

1. HOW DO YOU MEASURE BLOOD VOLUME?

⊃ A reliable method of measurement would be a considerable advance in medical science but regrettably it does not yet exist.

One technique uses a known volume of ^{51}Cr-radiolabelled red cells, which are injected into the circulation and allowed to equilibrate. A sample is taken later, and the blood volume may be calculated from:

Blood volume in ml $=$ $\dfrac{\text{Quantity of test substance injected}}{\text{Concentration of test substance observed}}$

Where the test substance is the labelled red cells.

An alternative technique involves the use of either radio-labelled albumin or Evans blue. Albumin will eventually distribute outside the vascular compartment, but initially it will reside in the plasma. The same mathematics is applied, but the measurement obtained is of course a measurement of plasma volume. In order to know the volume of blood, this equation is applied:

Blood volume in ml $=$ plasma volume $\times$ $\dfrac{100}{100 - \text{haematocrit}}$

2. WHAT IS THE EFFECT OF SEVERE HAEMORRHAGE ON PULMONARY FUNCTION?

⊃ Systematically approach this answer as follows:

1. Hyperventilation occurs secondary to the acidosis, which itself arises as a consequence of hypovolaemia and regional underperfusion.
2. Hypoxic pulmonary vasoconstriction will be seen, which is a paradox in this case, as it causes increased $\dot{V}/\dot{Q}$ mismatch and further deterioration in pulmonary function.

3. There is an increase in respiratory dead space.
4. Oxygen hunger-gasping deep respiration, represents a chemoreceptor response to hypotension.

3.   WHAT IS THE FICK PRINCIPLE?

> ⊃ The Fick principle states that the amount of a substance taken up by an organ (or by the whole body) per unit of time is equal to the arterial level of the substance minus the venous level multiplied by the blood flow. It can be employed to calculate blood flow, in the knowledge of the other variables, or to calculate $\dot{V}O_2$, oxygen consumption.

By taking simultaneous arterial and mixed venous samples it is possible to derive the difference in oxygen content. Mixed venous blood may be taken from the tip of a pulmonary artery (PA) catheter, or from a catheter in the right ventricle. Blood from the PA may contain shunted blood, however, which will lead to inaccuracies. Then:

$$\dot{Q} = \frac{\dot{V}O_2}{(CaO_2 - C\bar{v}O_2)}$$

For CaO_2 and $C\bar{v}O_2$:

O_2 content $= (1.31 \times Hb \times Saturation/100) + 0.002\, PO_2$

The $\dot{V}O_2$ can then be assessed in the light of the cardiac output at that time. A critically ill patient may require a $\dot{V}O_2$ 30% greater than normal.

4.   WHAT IS MIXED VENOUS OXYGEN SATURATION?

> ⊃ Mixed venous oxygen saturation is the percentage of mixed venous blood which is oxygenated, and may be measured photometrically at the tip of a Pulmonary Artery (PA) catheter.

$S\bar{v}O_2$ is decreased with:
1. Anaemia
2. Low cardiac output
3. Arterial oxygen desaturation
4. Increased oxygen consumption

$S\bar{v}O_2$ is increased with:
1. Sepsis associated with peripheral shunting
2. Cyanide toxicity
3. Hypothermia
4. Wedging of a PA catheter

5. WHAT ARE THE DETERMINANTS OF OXYGEN FLUX?

⊃ **Oxygen Flux = Cardiac output × Arterial oxygen content.**

O_2 content (ml/dl blood) = $(1.31^\star \times Hb \times Saturation/100) + 0.02\ PO_2$

$\star$ This is the oxygen content of one gram of haemoglobin molcule when fully saturated, the Hufner constant. The actual figure is quoted variously between 1.31 and 1.39 (ml O_2/g haemoglobin). 0.02 is the solubility coefficient of oxygen in blood at 37°C and is used to show the oxygen carried in solution in both erythrocyes and plasma (ml/dl per kPa). It is often quoted as an index, i.e. per m^2 of Body Surface Area (BSA).

6. WHAT CHANGES OCCUR IN RESPONSE TO TRAINING?

⊃ **Training results in a predictable pattern of multisystemic changes affecting the cardiovascular, respiratory and musculoskeletal systems.**

1. Maximal O_2 uptake increases. Maximal Breathing Capacity usually exceeds pulmonary ventilation at maximal exercise. The limiting factor is cardiac output and O_2 delivery; however O_2 diffusing capacity also increases.
2. Marathon runners can achieve a maximal Cardiac Output (CO) about 40% greater than untrained people. This occurs by an increase in heart muscle mass and an increase in heart size. End-diastolic volume and stroke volume both increase. This is why at rest the trained person has a lower heart rate than the untrained person.
3. There is an increase in muscle mass due to hypertrophy of individual muscle fibres, more storage of glycogen and proliferation of capillaries. The increased number of capillaries decreases intercapillary distance and allows improved blood supply during exercise. As a consequence O_2 debt only occurs later in exercise.

7. WHAT ARE THE FUNCTIONS OF PLATELETS?

⊃ **Platelets are formed from bone marrow megakaryocytes.**

Platelets have the following physiological roles:

1. In a platelet plug collagen contact causes ADP release which causes platelet activation.
2. Platelets are involved in histamine storage and release.
3. Thromboxanes cause platelet adhesion (cyclo-oxygenase function; arachidonic acid metabolism).
4. Platelet-derived growth factor (PDGF) stimulates wound healing and is a mitogen for vascular smooth muscle.

8. WHAT IS CONTRACTILITY AND HOW DO WE DETERMINE IT?

> ⊃ Contractility refers to the inotropic state of the heart independent of end-diastolic volume, heart rate and systemic vascular resistance.

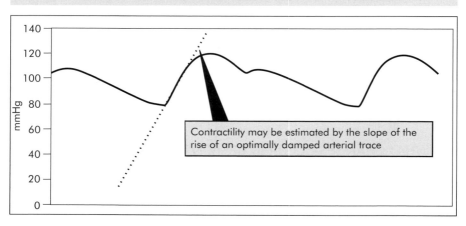

Contractility may be estimated by the slope of the rise of an optimally damped arterial trace

9. WHAT ARE THE FUNCTIONS OF LYMPH?

> ⊃ Questions on lymph may also concern composition as well as function.

1. To return interstitial fluid to the circulation as lymph. Lymphatic capillaries do not have tubes flowing into them, unlike blood capillaries. There are one-way valves governing the flow into the cisterna chyli from the lymphatic duct.
2. Lymph nodes are a focus of immune activity.
3. The total generated is 4L lymph/day, which acts to prevent the formation of oedema.
4. Lymphatics are responsible for the absorption of fat from intestine.

Composition of lymph is shown below:

Lymphatic fluid has:

- Lower protein content than plasma (varies with organ)
- Coagulation factors
- High levels of antibodies
- Similar electrolytic composition to plasma
- Lymphocytes in high number but few RBCs and platelets

10. DRAW THE PRESSURE CURVES FOR THE LEFT VENTRICLE AND AORTA

↻ **Expect the line of enquiry to concern timings and valve sequencing particularly.**

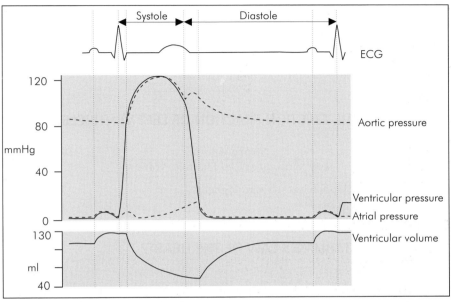

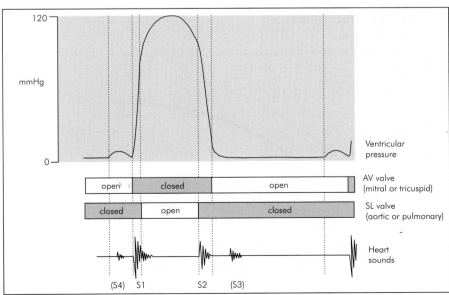

11. WHAT IS AUTOREGULATION OF BLOOD FLOW?

> ⊃ Autoregulation is the ability of an organ to control its blood supply
> independently of neural and hormonal influence. There are two main
> mechanisms whereby it is mediated.

1. A fall in arterial pressure results in a reduction in blood flow, and
   accumulation of metabolites; these cause local terminal arteriolar dilation,
   which in turn increases flow.
2. Myogenic response: This involves local neural reflexes in response to
   stretch, at the level of the 1st order arteriole.

12. WHAT IS THE EJECTION FRACTION OF LEFT VENTRICLE?

$$\text{Ejection fraction} = \frac{\text{Stroke Volume}}{\text{Left Ventricular End Diastolic Volume}}$$

■ Measure by Doppler at echocardiography
■ Normal >0.6. or 60%

13. WHAT IS STARLING'S LAW OF THE HEART?

> ⊃ Starling's law of the heart states that stroke volume is proportional to
> left ventricular end diastolic volume, to pressure, and to the length of
> the myofibril, therefore:

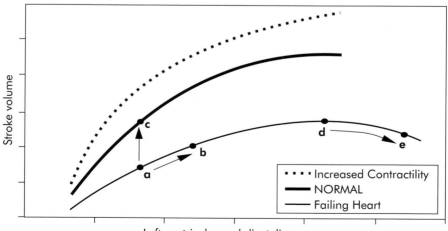

This change of output due to change in fibre length is also known as heterometric regulation, as opposed to homometric regulation which is change in output due to altered contractility. The implication of the shape of the curves is that the failing heart will generate less stroke volume for the same end-diastolic volume.

Starling originally stated that *"The energy of contraction [of a myofibril] is proportional to the initial length of the cardiac muscle fiber" (sic)*.

This has been extrapolated to imply that the stroke volume is proportional to the end diastolic volume. If the compliance of the heart is assumed to be constant then the stroke volume is proportional to the end diastolic pressure. If the mitral valve is functioning normally then the end diastolic pressure is the same as the left atrial pressure. The object of a pulmonary capillary wedge pressure reading is to record the pressure in the pulmonary venous system and therefore in the left atrium by using a static column of blood to transmit the pressure to the transducer. Therefore the stroke volume may be proportional to the pulmonary capillary wedge pressure.

Changes in the left ventricular end diastolic pressure ("preload") e.g. by altering the circulating volume, lead to shifts along one particular line (**a** to **b**), whereas changes in the contractility of the heart (e.g. by use of inotropic drugs) lead to a change of line (**a** to **c**). Therefore it can be seen that in the impaired myocardium a change in preload has a smaller effect than in the normal heart and can rapidly lead to the point where an increase in preload leads to a decrease in contractility (**d** to **e**).

---

14. WHAT ARE THE STARLING FORCES IN CAPILLARIES, AND WHAT HAPPENS TO THEM IF 500ML BLOOD IS LOST?

> ⊃ The forces are both hydrostatic and osmotic. You must be able to describe this diagram.

P_c Capillary hydrostatic pressure (varies from artery to vein)

P_{if} Interstitial hydrostatic pressure (usually 0)

π_p Oncotic pressure due to plasma proteins (28 mmHg)

π_{if} Oncotic pressure due to interstitial proteins (3 mmHg)

(Osmotic = hydrostatic and oncotic)

$$\text{Net filtration} = \underset{\uparrow}{(P_c} - \underset{\uparrow}{P_{if})} - \underset{\uparrow}{(\pi_p} - \underset{\uparrow}{\pi_{if})}$$

	varies	constant	constant	constant

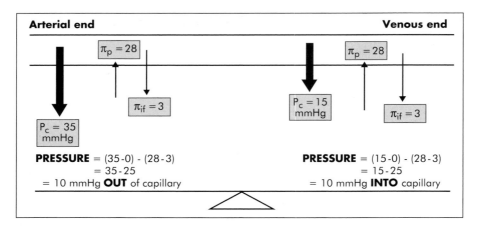

If the patient loses 500 ml of blood acutely, then the capillary hydrostatic pressure (P_c) falls especially at the venous end. The net pressure into the capillary increases and the balance is no longer maintained so fluid is retrieved into the circulation from the interstitium until P_c is restored. Note that this will also lead to small changes in π_p and π_{if}.

15. WHAT CARDIORESPIRATORY CHANGES OCCUR IN PREGNANCY?

⊃ **There are changes in the circulatory volume, the cardiac output, and the pattern and depth of respiration.**

1. Increased circulatory volume:
   - Increased red cell mass by 20% (an action of erythropoeitin)
   - Increased plasma volume by 50% (due to NaCl and water retention)

2. Increased cardiac output: by 60% at 28 weeks
   - Increase in heart rate by 15%
   - Increase in stroke volume by 30%
   - Reduced systemic vascular resistance, so creating a tendency to vascular engorgement
   - Mean arterial pressure stays constant
   - Increase in glomerular filtration rate by 50%

3. Increased ventilation: Alveolar ventilation increases by 70% at term.
   - Reduced $PaCO_2$
   - Increased tidal volume
   - Reduction in FRC by 20%

16. WHAT ARE THE CHANGES IN THE FOETAL CIRCULATION AT BIRTH?

> ⟳ The key is the change in pressures induced by the sudden change in pulmonary vascular resistance

Prior to birth:

Pulmonary vascular resistance is high because the lungs are not inflated. Blood from the right side of the heart, rather than go into the pulmonary arteries, goes into the ductus arteriosus and into the aorta, or through the foramen ovale and into the left atrium – because the pressure on the right side exceeds the pressure on the left.

At first gasp:

The lungs inflate and the pulmonary vascular resistance falls. There is suddenly a reduction in right-sided pressure and so the pressure on the left side now exceeds the pressure on the right.

As a result in the pressure change:

■ The foramen ovale closes.
■ Oxygenated blood flows retrograde in the ductus arteriosus.

As a result of this change:

■ The ductus arteriosus closes (but if cyanosed this fails to happen).

---

17. HOW DOES CORONARY BLOOD FLOW ALTER DURING THE CARDIAC CYCLE?

> ⟳ Coronary flow occurs in diastole (because intramyocardial vessels are compressed in systole) and is proportional to metabolic activity; in this way the system autoregulates.

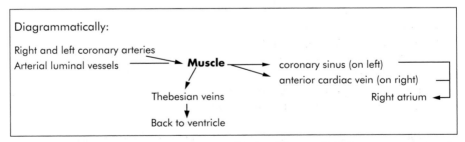

Diagrammatically:

Right and left coronary arteries
Arterial luminal vessels ⟶ **Muscle** ⟶ coronary sinus (on left)
anterior cardiac vein (on right) ⟶ Right atrium
Thebesian veins
↓
Back to ventricle

Coronary blood flow at rest is 250 ml/min. Myocardial O_2 consumption is 11 ml/100 g tissue/min (for skeletal muscle it is 8 ml/100 g tissue/min).

Coronary venous PO_2 is very low, so increased demand cannot be met by increased extraction – increased flow is required.

So: Increased heart rate → decreased diastolic time → decreased supply.

Increased intraventricular pressure → decreased supply.

The pressure compresses vessels, decreasing supply, which happens in hypertensives and is one reason why they are susceptible to myocardial ischaemia.

---

18. WHAT ARE PORTAL CIRCULATIONS?

> ⊃ A portal circulation is one that connects two capillary beds but does not receive a direct arterial supply nor drain into a venous system.

There are two of significance:

■ *The hepatic portal vein*, connecting the alimentary tract and the liver, conveys blood containing nutrients as well as toxins, and the liver converts the nutrients for storage or usage and metabolises the toxins. The hepatic portal circulation is vulnerable to a number of pathological processes, but if portal blood enters the systemic circulation, confusion, delirium or hepatic coma may ensue as toxins reach the central nervous system. In cirrhosis, portal hypertension may result, with distension of veins that form part of the circulation. Those that lie in the lower part of the oesophagus are vulnerable to trauma and represent a common source of upper gastro-intestinal bleeding.

■ *Hypothalamic – pituitary circulation* which conveys blood between the hypothalamus and the anterior pituitary. The arterial source is from the carotid arteries and the circle of Willis, which form the primary plexus on the ventral surface of the hypothalamus. Capillaries drain into vessels, which travel down the pituitary stalk and end in the pituitary capillaries. The hormones transiting this circulation are:

1. Thyrotropin releasing hormone (TRH)

2. Corticotropin releasing hormone (CRH)

3. Gonadotropin releasing hormone (GnRH)

4. Prolactin releasing hormone (PRH)

5. Prolactin inhibiting hormone (PIH)

6. Growth hormone releasing hormone (GRH)

7. Somatostatin

---

19. WHAT IS THE DISTINCTION BETWEEN THE HAEMOGLOBIN AND THE MYOGLOBIN OXYGEN DISSOCIATION CURVES?

⊃ The myoglobin oxygen dissociation curve lies to the left of the haemoglobin dissociation curve, which means that there is a tendency for haemoglobin to offload oxygen to myoglobin.

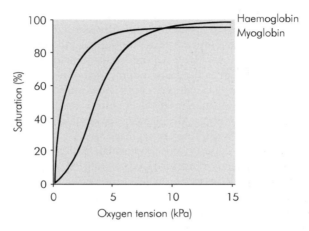

1. Oxygen binding to haemoglobin is co-operative
2. O_2 – haemoglobin affinity is pH dependant whereas O_2 – myoglobin is not
3. O_2 – haemoglobin affinity is affected by 2,3–DPG

The combined effect of the above means that haemoglobin has a lower affinity for O_2 than has myoglobin.

Expressed as a Hill plot:

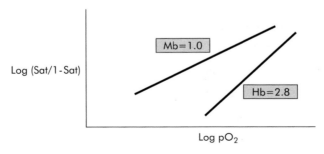

The fact that the Hill Coefficient for haemoglobin is greater than 1.0 means that the binding of O_2 to haemoglobin is co-operative.

So:

▨ Binding of O_2 at one tetramer facilitates binding at another
▨ Unloading of O_2 at one tetramer facilitates unloading at another

20. WHAT IS THE RESPONSE TO SUDDEN INCREASE IN ALTITUDE?

⊃ **This is about decompression at altitude. If sudden, this will be observed:**

- ▓ *Cold.* Temperature at 25,000 feet is usually -30°C. This is governed by the lapse rate, which is a drop in temperature of 1.98°C/1,000 feet.
- ▓ *Misting.* This is because of the dew point. There is an upper limit to the amount of water vapour air can hold at any temperature; when this maximum is reached the air is said to be saturated. Saturated air at high temperatures holds more water vapour than saturated air at low temperatures. The temperature at saturation is called the dew point. When decompression occurs, there is a sudden drop in temperature, but the same percentage of the air in the cabin is composed of water vapour, (even though the absolute quantity is reduced – but for the purposes of humidity it is percentages which matter) so the dew point is reached, and misting occurs.
- ▓ *Hypoxia if above 8,000 feet.* Alveolar air very rapidly equilibrates with the new ambient conditions. Pulmonary capillary blood will actually yield oxygen to the alveoli, in the opposite sense to normal, further accelerating the problem. This means that arterial oxygen tension falls very rapidly, depending on the severity of the decompression, with similarly rapid onset of symptoms of hypoxia.
- ▓ *Expansion of closed cavities*, because decreased pressure leads to increased volume.

The clinical observation is of a lowering in PaO_2, with a simultaneous lowering of $PaCO_2$; this latter effect is because there is a need to hyperventilate to reduce CO_2 to "make room" for O_2 because:

$$P_AO_2 = P_IO_2 - \frac{P_ACO_2}{R}$$

This contrasts with the effect of breathing a hypoxic gas mixture, which would be a question about the normal hypercapnia drive to ventilation and the fact that confusion, discoordination and ultimately unconsciousness occur before any profound dyspnoea is evident.

___

21. WHAT IS THE PHYSIOLOGICAL RESPONSE TO HAEMORRHAGE?

⊃ Consider the four different interlinked systems: cardiovascular response, pituitary response, renin–aldosterone–angiotensin, and endocrine response from sympathetic nervous system.

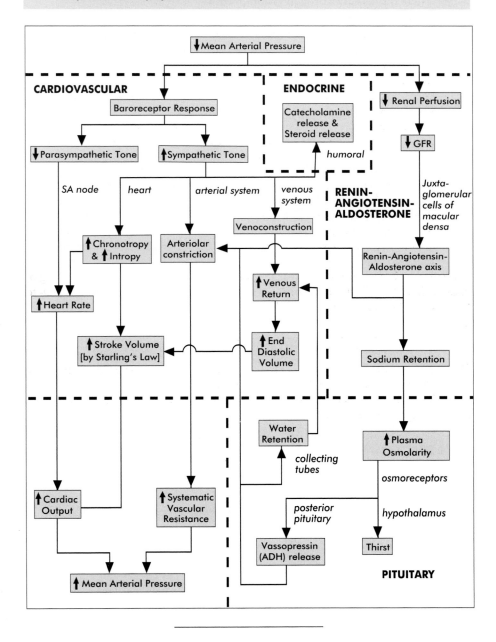

22. DESCRIBE THE VALSALVA MANOEUVRE?

> ⊃ **The Valsalva manoeuvre is forced expiration against a closed glottis**

- There is an increase in intrathoracic pressure
- There is therefore a drop in venous return

The normal person maintains mean arterial pressure by:

- Increasing heart rate
- Increasing systemic vascular resistance
- And demonstrates, on release, transient hypertension and bradycardia

There are four phases which can be drawn in a diagram:

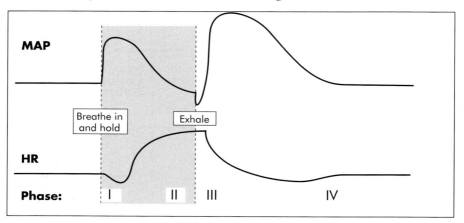

Phase I: The increase in intrathoracic pressure adds to arterial pressure producing a rise in mean arterial pressure.

Phase II: The mean arterial pressure then falls because of reduced venous return.

Phase III: On releasing, there is an overshoot as vasoconstriction and an increase in heart rate are still in operation.

Phase IV: Return to normal.

The normal Valsalva response is absent or abnormal in autonomic dysfunction, in particular autonomic neuropathy (in diabetes mellitus, for example) and after sympathectomy.

23. CAN YOU DRAW THE CARDIAC ACTION POTENTIAL?

⊃ At rest, the membrane is more permeable to K⁺ than Na⁺ thus the potential difference (Nernst equation) applies more to K⁺ (–90 mV) than to Na⁺ (+60 mV).

⊃ It is the continuation of depolarisation which distinguishes cardiac action potential (AP) from skeletal AP. This is due to the action of slow Ca^{2+} channels, allowing Ca^{2+} entry into the cell, maintaining a balance against K⁺ outwards, so causing a prolonged depolarisation.

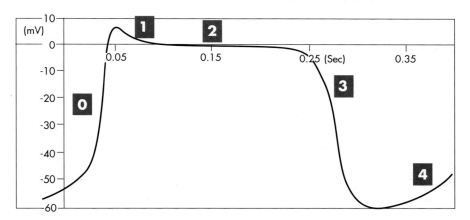

Phase:

    0 = Fast depolarisation, Na^+ inwards
    1 = Early incomplete repolarisation
    2 = Plateau, slow Ca^{2+} inwards, prolonging AP
    3 = Rapid repolarisation, K^+ outwards
    4 = Electrical diastole, refractory period

Ca^{2+} is functionally related to β-receptors
K^+ is functionally related to M_2 receptors and β-receptors
Changes in external K^+ affect the resting potential level
Changes in internal Na^+ affect the magnitude of the action potential

Effects on rate of firing:

Acetylcholine works at muscarinic (M_2) receptors, causing increased K^+ permeability (especially at K^+ channels), which in turn causes hyperpolarisation and decreased rate of firing.

Norepinephrine acts at β receptors to cause decreased K^+ permeability and increased rate of firing. It also acts at β receptors causing increased Ca^{2+} permeability and increased strength of contraction.

24. WHAT ARE THE CAROTID BODIES AND SINUSES AND THEIR DIFFERENCES?

⊃ **The carotid bodies respond to oxygen tension; the carotid sinus is a baroreceptor.**

Carotid (and aortic) bodies:
Contain two types of cell which are sensitive to OXYGEN

- Type I (Glomus) cells – adjacent to unmyelinated nerve endings from Glossopharyngeal nerve (IX). Dopamine exerts an inhibitory effect.
- Type II – sustentacular cells.

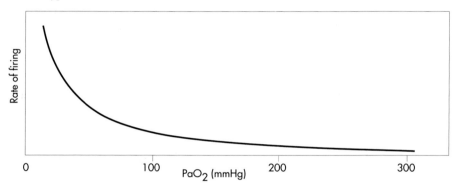

Carotid bodies receive a colossal arterial blood supply: 2 litres/100 g tissue/minute. This means the glomus cells can function on supply from dissolved oxygen alone, and are unaffected by anaemia or CO poisoning.

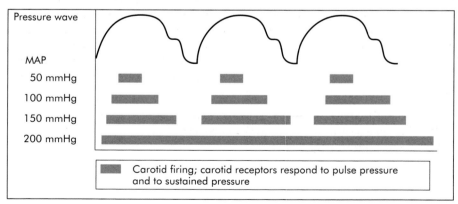

Carotid Sinus:
This is situated at a dilatation of the internal carotid at its bifurcation, and responds to **PRESSURE**. Baroreceptors in dilatation resemble golgi tendon organs. The carotid sinus nerve is a branch of the glossopharyngeal (IX).

25. WHAT IS ARTERIO-VENOUS O_2 DIFFERENCE?

> ⊃ This is the difference in oxygen tension between the arterial and venous circulations, reflecting the oxygen consumption of an organ or of the whole body.

- ▦ O_2 content $= 1.31 \times (Hb \times Sat/100) + 0.02\ PaO_2$
- ▦ SvO_2 may be measured by a photometric cell at the pulmonary artery catheter tip (and thus $C\bar{v}O_2$ may be calculated from the above)
- ▦ PaO_2 can be measured directly from an arterial sample, and arterial O_2 calculated as above
- ▦ Q, cardiac output, may be obtained from calorimetric measurement

This allows calculation of $\dot{V}O_2$, oxygen consumption, from:

$$\text{Fick} \quad \dot{Q} \quad = \quad \frac{\dot{V}O_2}{CaO_2 - C\bar{v}O2}$$

Diminished $\dot{V}O_2$ is the earliest pathophysiological event in shock, and usually precedes the hypotension that characterises it.

---

26. WHAT FACTORS MODIFY DIASTOLIC BLOOD PRESSURE?

> ⊃ Diastolic blood pressure is principally determined by cardiovascular afterload.

Whereas systolic blood pressure is related to myocardial contractility and to ventricular filling, diastolic blood pressure is related to afterload. Therefore, systemic vascular resistance is a major contributor to diastolic blood pressure. For example, in patent ductus arteriosus of the new born, diastolic pressure maybe unmeasurable until the patent ductus is surgically ligated, in which case diastolic pressure becomes measurable. Diastolic pressure, itself is a determinant of coronary artery filling and both duration of diastole and diastolic blood pressure have a bearing on the adequacy of coronary perfusion.

Certain valvular heart conditions, notably aortic regurgitation, will produce a widened pulse pressure and a diminished diastolic blood pressure. This may have implications for coronary perfusion.

---

27. DRAW THE CARDIAC PACEMAKER CELL ACTION POTENTIAL. WHAT ALTERS ITS DURATION?

⊃ The action potential produced when a pacemaker cell depolarises is a slow response type AP, which is classified into phases (0–4). Phase 1, the rapid repolarisation phase is a characteristic of the myocyte AP rather than a pacemaker cell and phase 2 is extremely brief.

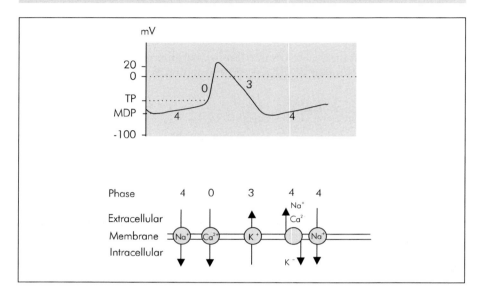

Pacemaker cells show inherent rhythmicity due to a spontaneous depolarisation from –60 mV to about –40 mV. In this so-called phase 4, sodium and calcium ions leak into the cell and this is not balanced by the egress of potassium ions (down the concentration gradient). There thus develops a prepotential also known as pacemaker potential. When a certain threshold is reached (-40 mV), Calcium channels open resulting in rapid depolarisation. Repolarisation in phase 3 occurs due to the egress of potassium ions.

This contrasts to nerve action potential where the upstroke of the action potential is due to opening of (rapid) sodium channels.

Heart rate is altered by slope of prepotential, which is affected by the following:

Sympathetic system: Norepinephrine causes more rapid opening of calcium channels. This is achieved by Norepinephrine binding β receptors which increase cAMP that cause calcium channels to open

Parasympathetic nervous system: Acetylcholine increases potassium permeability of pacemaker membrane and allows more potassium to flow OUT of cell. Therefore the cell is more negative. This reduces rate of calcium channel opening.

Temperature: Cold decreases the slope of the prepotential causing slower depolarisation.

> ⊃ **Differences between the pacemaker and myocyte action potential:**

Pacemaker has:
- Less negative phase 4 membrane potential
- Less negative threshold potential
- Spontaneous depolarisation in phase 4
- Less steep slope in phase 0
- Absence of phase 2 (plateau)

---

28. WHAT IS OEDEMA? WHAT ARE THE CAUSES OF OEDEMA?

> ⊃ **Oedema is the accumulation of interstitial fluid in abnormally large amounts.**

Mechanism involves:
- Starling Forces
- Rise in capillary pressure above oncotic pressure throughout the length of the capillary
- Accumulation of osmotically active metabolites in interstitium that are not so quickly washed away exerts osmotic gradient

Fluid movement $= k[(P_c + \pi_i) - (P_i + \pi_c)]$

k = capillary filtration coefficient

P_c = capillary hydrostatic pressure

P_i = interstitial hydrostatic pressure

π_c = capillary colloid osmotic pressure

π_i = interstitial colloid osmotic pressure

Causes of increased interstitial fluid volume and oedema:
Increased capillary pressure

- Arteriolar dilatation
- Venular constriction
- Increased venous pressure (heart failure, incompetent valves, venous obstruction, gravity)

Decreased osmotic pressure gradient

- Decrease plasma proteins, for example renal failure, decreased albumin seen in critically ill

Increase in capillary permeability

- Substance P, Kinins, Histamine

Inadequate lymph flow

- Obstruction example by tumours, radical mastectomy

3

QUESTIONS IN RESPIRATORY PHYSIOLOGY

1. CAN YOU DRAW THE OXYHAEMOGLOBIN DISSOCIATION CURVE?

⊃ **If you cannot draw an accurate curve and mark on the three most relevant points you will be likely to gain a 1 mark.**

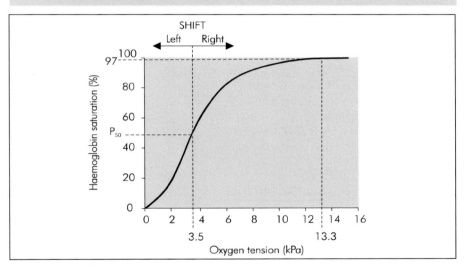

Arterial	97% saturated	PO_2 13.3 kPa
Mixed venous	75% saturated	PO_2 5.3kPa
P_{50}	50% saturated	PO_2 3.5 kPa

The P_{50} allows comparison between situations with respect to shift of the curve. Remember that right shift is caused by **increases** and *vice versa*. Thus right shift occurs in:

 Acidosis (increased hydrogen ions)
 Increased PCO_2
 Increased 2,3-DPG
 Increased temperature

2. CAN YOU DERIVE THE BOHR EQUATION?

> ⊃ The Bohr equation allows derivation of total (physiological) dead space.
> Mistakes in derivation will not fail you. Ignorance of the underlying
> relevance of the principle involved will.

1. $V_{D\,Phys} = V_{D\,Anat} + V_{D\,Alv}$
2. V_A = volume of alveoli. F_ACO_2 = Fraction of alveolar gas that is CO_2
   V_D = volume of dead space. F_ECO_2 = Fraction of expired gas that is CO_2
   Tidal Volume, $V_T = V_D + V_A$
3. All CO_2 comes from alveoli (V_A) and none from dead space (V_D).
   (Like the shunt equation, use total gas expired).
   $V_T \times F_ECO_2$ = total CO_2 "Flux" by analogy; collect in bag and measure
   Which all comes from $V_A \times F_ACO_2$
4. $V_T = V_A + V_D$
   Therefore $V_A = V_T - V_D$
5. Substitute 3 into 4.
   $V_T \times F_ECO_2 = (V_T - V_D) \times F_ACO_2$
6. Expand
   $V_T \times F_ECO_2 = (V_T \times F_ACO_2) - (V_D \times F_ACO_2)$
7. Add, so as to get VT on one side
   $V_D \times F_ACO_2 = (V_T \times F_ACO_2) - (V_T - F_ECO_2)$
8. Simplify right side
   $V_D \times F_ACO_2 = V_T \times (F_ACO_2 - F_ECO_2)$
9. Rearrange
   $$V_D/V_T = \frac{F_ACO_2 - F_ECO_2}{F_ACO_2}$$
10. Bohr $$\frac{V_D}{V_T} = \frac{P_ACO_2 - P_ECO_2}{P_ACO2}$$

---

3. HOW DO YOU MEASURE RESPIRATORY DEAD SPACE?

> ⊃ Dead space is that part of inspired gas which does not take part in gas
> exchange. It is divided into alveolar dead space, $V_{D\,alv}$, which consists of
> unperfused alveoli, and anatomical dead space, $V_{D\,anat}$, which consists of
> the conducting airways.

Helium dilution allows measurement of TOTAL LUNG CAPACITY, from which
you can derive residual volume and FRC, by using spirometry and arithmetic.
However it cannot measure that volume which is behind closed airways, because the
Helium cannot get there; so:

In order to measure FRC in, for example, a patient with emphysema and airway closure, the body plethysmograph must be used. This uses Boyle's law, $P1 \times V1 = P2 \times V2$.

Anatomical dead space can be measured by Fowler's method, slow exhalation after single breath of 100% O_2, monitoring Nitrogen concentration. A perpendicular through phase II locates $V_{D\,anat}$. The dead space is the volume up to the vertical line, placed so that the areas A and B are equal.

$$V_{D\,phys} = V_{D\,alv} + V_{D\,anat}$$

For $V_{D\,phys}$, use the Bohr equation: $\quad \dfrac{V_D}{V_T} \quad = \quad \dfrac{P_ACO_2 - P_ECO_2}{P_ACO_2}$

For $V_{D\,anat}$, Single breath O_2

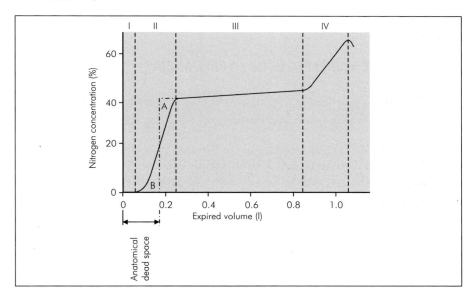

4.   WHAT IS RESPIRATORY QUOTIENT (RQ)?

> ⊃ This is the ratio *in steady state* of the volume of carbon dioxide
> produced to the volume of oxygen consumed per unit time.

The respiratory quotient is *not* the same as **respiratory exchange ratio (R)**, which
is the ratio of CO_2 to O_2 at ANY time.

Therefore $RQ = \dfrac{CO_2 \text{ produced at equilibrium}}{O_2 \text{ consumed}}$

> ⊃ What happens to the RQ if the patient is given an opioid such as Fentanyl?

RQ decreases as hypoventilation will result in decreased CO_2 measured at the
mouth.

5.   WHAT ARE THE EFFECTS OF HYPERCARBIA?

> ⊃ Hypercarbia is defined as a $PaCO_2$ greater than 45 mmHg (6.0 kPa). You
> should divide your answer into discussion of effects on each system in turn.

- Effects on the central nervous system: Elevated $PaCO_2$ raises cerebral blood
  flow due to increased $[H^+]$. This effect only lasts until bicarbonate buffering
  becomes effective, at about 24 – 48 hours. Hypercarbia stimulates the
  sympathetic nervous system.
- Effects on the respiratory system: Elevation of $PaCO_2$ up to 13.0 kPa
  stimulates respiration, beyond that point it is a respiratory depressant. It also
  increases pulmonary vascular resistance.

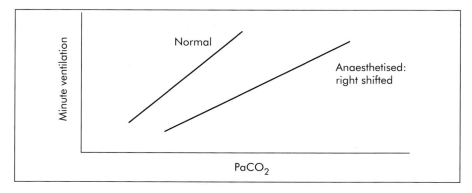

- Effects on the cardiovascular system: Carbon dioxide is a direct myocardial
  depressant and a potent vasodilator. This effect is blunted at modest levels of
  hypercarbia because of the consequent sympathetic stimulation; more
  severe rises result in a fall in cardiac output and arterial pressure.

6. WHAT FACTORS AFFECT PULMONARY VASCULAR RESISTANCE?

> ⊃ Consider both those factors which increase pulmonary vascular resistance (PVR) and those which reduce it.

Factors increasing pulmonary vascular resistance:
- A reduction in alveolar PO_2, which is known as hypoxic pulmonary vasoconstriction. This is a protective mechanism, which should divert blood away from locally under-ventilated areas. The effect is probably mediated by a fall in nitric oxide (NO)
- A rise in CO_2 concentration and acidosis
- Epinephrine, dopamine, histamine, 5-HT
- Lung collapse

Factors reducing pulmonary vascular resistance:
- Increased cardiac output by recruitment of capillaries
- Acetylcholine and cholinergics, possibly also an NO effect
- Isoprenaline
- Prostacyclin

---

7. HERE IS AN ARTERIAL BLOOD GAS SAMPLE, SHOWING ELEVATED CO_2 WITH LOW O_2. CAN YOU INTERPRET IT?

> ⊃ You may be given a blood gas result to comment on. Several pictures may be shown. Make sure you know which measurements of a blood-gas analyser are direct and which are derived. Be able to define a 'standard' value (sample titrated to PCO_2 of 5.3 kPa).

High CO_2 with low O_2 implies type II respiratory failure: an exhausted asthmatic, for example.

- PCO_2 is related to ventilatory function and minute ventilation
- PO_2 is related to gas exchange and inspired oxygen fraction

Low pH and low PO_2 implies tissue acidosis. It is possible to differentiate acute from chronic hypoventilation by pH;

- Acute = acidotic, **NORMAL** bicarbonate
- Compensated = normal pH, **HIGH** bicarbonate

---

8. WHAT IS THE ALVEOLAR – ARTERIAL O_2 GRADIENT?

> ⊃ **This is the difference between the observed arterial O_2 content and the calculated ideal alveolar O_2 content.**

It may be calculated by subtracting the arterial PO_2 (measured) from the ideal alveolar PO_2, which may be calculated from:

$$P_AO_2 \quad = \quad P_IO_2 \ - \ \frac{P_ACO_2}{R}$$

The gradient is normally less than 2 kPa and is increased in disease states:

1. Right to left vascular shunt
2. Ventilation/perfusion defects
3. Diffusion impairment: extravascular lung water, pulmonary fibrosis, etc.
4. Adult respiratory distress syndrome
5. Neonatal respiratory distress syndrome

9. WHAT IS THE OXYGEN CASCADE?

> ⊃ **The oxygen cascade describes the drop in oxygen tension between atmospheric air and the surface of the mitochondrion.**

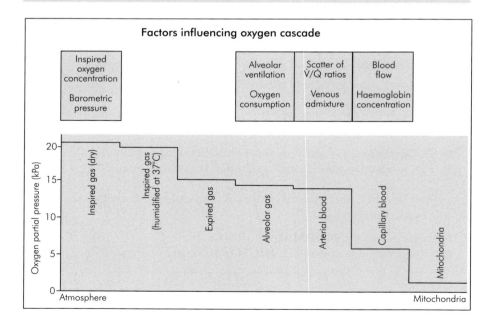

10.   WHAT IS PULMONARY VENOUS ADMIXTURE?

> ⊃ **Venous admixture equals true shunt plus $\dot{V}/\dot{Q}$ mismatch.**

From the 'shunt' equation $\dfrac{\dot{Q}s}{\dot{Q}T} = \dfrac{CiO_2 - CaO_2}{CiO_2 - C\bar{v}O_2}$

$\dot{Q}s/\dot{Q}T$ is the ratio of 'shunt' to total cardiac output

- CaO_2 ⎫ require arterial and mixed venous samples (from a
- $C\bar{v}O_2$ ⎬ pulmonary artery catheter) and this calculation:

O_2 content = (1.31 × Hb × Saturation/100) + 0.02 PO_2

True shunt:

- This is due to bronchial blood flow emerging from the bronchial veins; it represents 5% of cardiac output in normal states.

$\dot{V}/\dot{Q}$ mismatch: this is about the West zones.

- Apices are ventilated better than perfused;
- Midzones "normal", i.e. $P_a > P_A > P_v$
- Bases perfused better than ventilated.
- When $P_A > P_a > P_v$ (apices) there is no perfusion.

Ratio of V: Q totals at 1.0 : 0.8

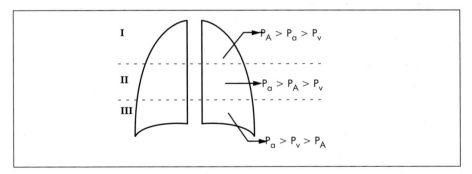

---

11. WHAT NON–RESPIRATORY FUNCTIONS OF THE LUNGS DO YOU KNOW?

1. Removal of vasoactive amines and neurotransmitters, which is a function of pulmonary endothelial cells.
2. Metabolism of Angiotensin I to Angiotensin II, which is a vasopressor and a part of the stress response.
3. Filtration of peripheral venous blood of clots, etc.
4. Phospholipid synthesis, e.g. dipalmitoyl phosphatidyl choline which is a component of surfactant.
5. Prostaglandin inactivation.
6. Leukotriene synthesis (from arachidonic acid, which is lipoxygenase mediated).
7. Immunoglobulin synthesis; IgA.

---

12. CAN YOU DRAW THE VOLUMES AND CAPACITIES OF THE LUNG?

> ↻ A capacity consists of TWO or more volumes.

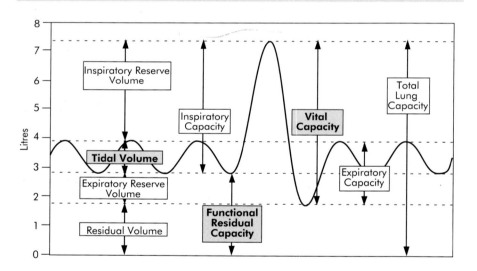

All figures refer to the adult.

Tidal volume: The volume of gas in a normal resting respiration. (500 ml or 7 ml/kg).

Vital capacity: The maximum amount of gas which can be used in one breath, made up of IRV and ERV in addition to TV.(4.5 l).

Total lung capacity: 7.5 l.

Functional residual capacity: An area of respiratory physiology of supreme interest to anaesthetists. This is the amount of gas in the lungs after a normal tidal breath. It is where the gas is exchanged, and is reduced by anaesthesia.

Closing Capacity = Closing Volume + Residual Volume: Closing Capacity is the volume of the lungs at which small airways start to close and rises with age. FRC is reduced by 20% in anaesthesia due to diaphragmatic shift, decreased ribcage dimensions and IPPV. If FRC falls below Closing Capacity, areas will be perfused but not ventilated.

13. HOW ARE THE ALVEOLAR PARTIAL PRESSURES OF CO_2 AND O_2 RELATED?

⊃ **The $O_2 - CO_2$ diagram shows the ventilation–perfusion ratio line.**

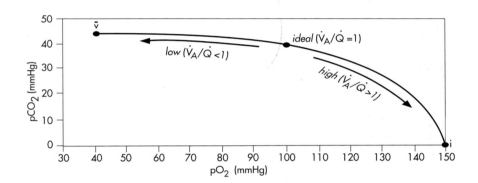

The oxygen and CO_2 composition of the blood are not independent, but related by means of this line. This shows all possible alveolar gas compositions for a lung with inspired fraction of 1, and the effects of increased and decreased $\dot{V}/\dot{Q}$ ratios.

14. CAN YOU DESCRIBE THE RISE IN P_AO_2 WHEN BREATHING 100% O_2?

> ⊃ This is about preoxygenation (denitrogenation), and the fact that the SVP of water vapour, 47 mmHg, applies to alveolar gas. It is independent of atmospheric pressure but does depend on temperature. It is NOT the same as the time taken for the SpO_2 to reach 100%.

For the whole body to be denitrogenated, the process proceeds at an exponential rate and takes several hours.

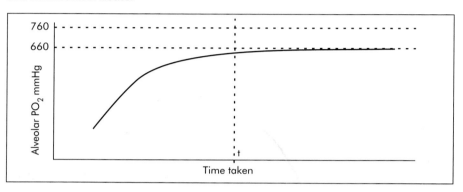

t, the time taken to equilibrium, is normally 10 minutes, but is affected by:

1. Health
2. Chronic airways disease, which increases t
3. Cardiac output, where a low output increases t

Most would advocate preoxygenation for 3–5 minutes, or for three vital capacity breaths. Water vapour occupies 47 mmHg and CO_2 40 mmHg, hence optimal alveolar O_2 at normal ventilation breathing 100% O_2 is around 660 mmHg.

$$P_AO_2 = P_IO_2 - \frac{P_aCO_2}{R}$$

$$= 1.0(760 - 47) - \frac{40}{0.8}$$

15. WHAT IS COMPLIANCE?

> ⊃ **Compliance is the change in volume per unit change in pressure.**

$$1/c_{\text{TOTAL}} = 1/c_{\text{LUNG}} + 1/c_{\text{CHEST WALL}}$$

Why reciprocals? Because pressure at a given volume is inversely proportional to compliance.

Compliance decreases with

- Venous congestion
- Oedema
- Intermittent positive pressure ventilation
- Fibrosis, emphysema
- Age

---

16. CAN YOU DESCRIBE RESPIRATION IN THE NEONATE?

> ⊃ **This can be divided into anatomical and physiological considerations.**

Anatomical:
- Neonates have a large head, a short neck, and a proportionally large tongue
- They have narrow passages
- They are nasal breathers; the epiglottis touches the soft palate
- Their larynx is high, and narrowest at the cricoid, which is at the level of C3–4
- The epiglottis is bigger in proportion, and it is U-shaped
- There is a wider carina than in older children, and both main bronchi are at equal angles
- There are 21 generations of airway
- There are 10% of the numbers of adult alveoli

Physiological:
- High compliance, small functional residual capacity (FRC)
- The closing volume added to the residual volume = closing capacity (CC); CC is greater than FRC until aged 5, which implies a tendency to airway closure and $\dot{V}/\dot{Q}$ mismatch
- Tidal volume is fixed because of:
  - ☐ Horizontal ribs
  - ☐ Weak intercostal muscles
  - ☐ Large abdomen

So, in order to increase minute volume ($\dot{V}E$), neonates need to increase respiratory rate (which is analogous to the situation with cardiac output in the neonate, where stroke volume is fixed, and rate dictates output).

- Respiratory rate is 32 breaths per minute in the neonate; to calculate aged 1–13, = (24-age/2) per minute
- Minute volume ~ 200 ml/kg body weight
- Tidal volume ~ 8 ml/kg body weight
- A low PaO_2, and a low $PaCO_2$ are compatible with normality
- There is no expiratory pause: The respiratory cycle is a sine wave

So for a 3 kg neonate:
$\dot{V}E$ = 600 ml
Tidal volume (V_T) = 20 ml

---

17. HOW IS ALVEOLAR VENTILATION CONTROLLED?

⊃ **Alveolar ventilation is proportional to rate of respiration and to depth of respiration.**

⊃ **Discuss receptors, comparators, and effectors.**

Receptors: Those responding to CO_2 are the most significant in health.

1. Receptors for $PaCO_2$ are present in the ventrolateral medulla near the IXth and Xth cranial nerves. These receptors are surrounded by cerebrospinal fluid (CSF) and are responsive to $[H^+]$ ion concentration and therefore indirectly to the presence of CO_2 by means of the action of carbonic anhydrase. The CO_2 diffuses across the blood brain barrier, $[H^+]$ is generated and the receptors stimulated. CSF has fewer proteins than plasma, and hence less buffering ability – so pH changes are more pronounced.

2. The receptors for PaO_2 are the carotid and aortic bodies. The type I glomus cells demonstrate a linear response to $[H^+]$; they respond to $[O_2]$ in a non-linear fashion, firing only when the PaO_2 falls below 13 kPa. The carotid and aortic bodies receive an abundant blood supply, which allows for precise comparisons to be made as they have a very low arterio-venous O_2 difference despite having a high metabolic rate. They are relatively indifferent to $PaCO_2$.

3. Airway stretch receptors: These act to terminate respiration, by means of the Hering-Breuer reflex.

4. Epithelial receptors in the larynx: These respond to irritants and inhibit respiration.

5. J Receptors (meaning juxta-capillary) respond to capillary engorgement (as in pulmonary oedema) by inhibiting respiration. This may be an explanation for the dypnoea of pulmonary oedema.

Comparators: These are all under a degree of control by the cortex

1. The Nucleus Parabrachialis Medialis (NPBM) is located in the pons and is referred to as the pneumotactic centre. It fine-tunes respiration, influencing the other centres which are lower in the brainstem.

2. The inspiratory centre may be responsible for the intrinsic pattern of respiration.

3. The expiratory centre is only active during exercise, as it is only then that expiration becomes important; it is otherwise passive.

Effectors:
1. Diaphragm: Inspiratory function predominates, under phrenic innervation.
2. Intercostals: These are expiratory in function.
3. Accessory muscles: These are only used in extreme situations.

---

18. HOW IS CO_2 TRANSPORTED IN THE BLOOD?

1. 60% as $HCO_3^- + H^+$ by means of carbonic anhydrase
2. 30% as $HbCO_2$
3. 10% dissolved in plasma

Resting production of CO_2 is 200 ml/minute.

$$\text{Respiratory quotient} \quad = \quad \frac{CO_2 \text{ produced}}{O_2 \text{ consumed}}$$

usually $\qquad = \qquad 0.8$

In Hb, combines with amino group

$$\text{R-NH}_2 \quad + \quad CO_2 \quad \rightarrow \quad \underset{\overset{|}{\text{H}}}{\text{R-N-COOH}}$$

Deoxyhaemoglobin has a higher affinity for both H^+ and CO_2 than does oxyhaemoglobin. This is the Haldane effect; thus O_2 deficient cells are better buffers than are oxygenated cells.

---

19. CAN YOU CLASSIFY HYPOXIA?

> ⟳ Hypoxia may be hypoxaemic, stagnant, cytotoxic or anaemic; after giving this definition, a discussion will follow on one of the four.

1. **Hypoxaemic hypoxia;** where the PaO_2 is reduced, which may be due to:
   - Hypoventilation
   - Diffusion impairment
   - Shunt
   - $\dot{V}/\dot{Q}$ mismatch (N.B. not deadspace which is to do with CO_2)
2. **Stagnant hypoxia;** where the blood supply to an organ is inadequate, even though the PaO_2 and the Hb concentration may be normal.
3. **Cytotoxic hypoxia;** where the oxygen delivery is normal, but the cell is prevented from utilising it, for example, cytochrome poisoning.
4. **Anaemic hypoxia;** where the PaO_2 is normal but the Hb concentration, and therefore the amount of O_2 delivered, is deficient.

---

20. WHAT IS THE WORK OF BREATHING?

> ⊃ **This is the work required to move the lung and chest wall.**

Work = pressure × volume. So, we need a pressure-volume curve to describe this phenomenon.

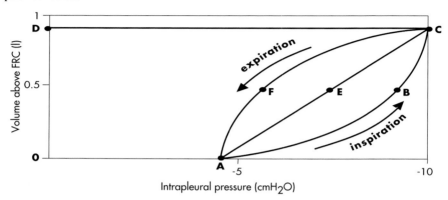

1. In inspiration the lung follows the line **ABC** and so the work done is described by the area **OABCDO** which is made up of:
   - **OAECDO** is the work required to overcome the elastic forces.
   - **ABCEA** is the work required to overcome the viscous (airway and tissue) resistance.
2. In expiration the area **AECFA** represents the work to overcome the airway (and tissue) resistance, and as this is within the area **OABCDO** it is accomplished by the stored energy within the elastic recoil that is released during passive expiration. The remaining part of the stored energy **OAFCDO**) is lost as heat. In states of higher airway resistance or higher inspiratory flow rate ABC curves more to the right (that is there is a greater negative intrapleural pressure for a given volume) thus the viscous volume **ABCEA** is larger. Thus at higher ventilatory rates the viscous work of breathing is increased.

However with larger tidal volumes the elastic work area **OAECDO** is increased. In patients with stiff lungs (thus reduced compliance) the elastic work is reduced by breathing with small tidal volumes at high respiratory rates (the so called 'pink puffer'), whereas in those patients with obstructive airway disease the viscous work is reduced by using a low respiratory rate, this the patients naturally find the respiratory pattern that ensures the lowest work of breathing.

$$\text{Efficiency} = \frac{\text{Useful work}}{\text{Energy expended}} \times 100$$

The efficiency of the work of breathing is usually about 5%; 5% is also the percentage of total O_2 consumption, at rest, used in the work of breathing.

21. WHAT IS THE HENDERSON–HASSELBALCH EQUATION?

> ⊃ **A buffer consists of weak acid with the conjugate base.**

$$H^+ + A^- \underset{k_2}{\overset{k_1}{\Leftrightarrow}} HA \text{ at equilibrium, } k_1 = k_2$$

$$\frac{[H^+] \times [A^-]}{[HA]} = K \text{ by the law of mass action}$$

$$pH = pK + \log \frac{[HCO_3^-]}{0.2\, PCO_2} \quad \text{where 0.2 is the solubility coefficient of } CO_2 \text{ in} \\ \text{mmol/l/kPa.}$$

It may usefully be simplified:

$$pH \propto \frac{[HCO_3^-]}{[CO_2]}$$

Such that if the bicarbonate rises, or the CO_2 falls, then the pH will rise (an alkalosis will develop); by the same token, if the bicarbonate falls, or the CO_2 rises, the pH will fall; this is an acidosis.

---

22. CAN YOU DERIVE THE SHUNT EQUATION?

> ⊃ **Need a diagram to do this.**

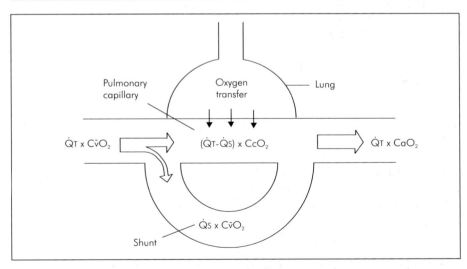

$$\dot{Q}T \times CaO_2 \quad = \quad \text{total oxygen flux from entire system}$$
$$= \quad \text{that via shunt + that via alveolar capillary}$$

$$= \dot{Q}S \times C\bar{v}O_2 \text{ (that blood which doesn't get oxygenated at all)}$$

$$+ (\dot{Q}T\text{-}\dot{Q}s) \times CcO_2$$

Thus: $\dot{Q}T \times CaO_2 = \dot{Q}S \times C\bar{v}O_2 + (\dot{Q}T - \dot{Q}S) \times CcO_2$

Rearranging $\dfrac{\dot{Q}S}{\dot{Q}T} = \dfrac{CcO_2 - CaO_2}{CcO_2 - C\bar{v}O_2}$

or $\dfrac{\dot{Q}S}{\dot{Q}T} = \dfrac{C_iO_2 - CaO_2}{C_iO_2 - C\bar{v}O_2}$ (C_iO_2 is obtained from alveolar gas equation)

---

23. DESCRIBE THE ACCLIMATISATION TO ASCENT TO 500 METRES.

⊃ **This may appear with various wording. The essential point is that hypoxia develops at altitude due to the atmosphere becoming 'thinner' as atmospheric pressure falls. The SVP of water vapour is a constant and thus takes up a proportionally bigger fraction of the inspired mixture.**

Initially respiratory alkalosis develops due to hyperventilation. The left shift of the ODC is exceeded by an increase in 2,3-DPG and the net result is a *small* increase in P_{50} (right shift). Ventilation increases further over a few days and then falls back, remaining at an increased level over normal for some years. Erythropoetin secretion rises and there is thus an increase in red cell mass.

Chronic changes include an increase in mitochondrial numbers, an increase in myoglobin concentration and higher levels of cytochrome oxidase.

4

QUESTIONS IN ENDOCRINE PHYSIOLOGY

1. WHAT ARE THE FUNCTIONS OF THE POSTERIOR PITUITARY?

> ⊃ The posterior pituitary produces hormones that influence plasma osmolarity and circulating volume, milk ejection and uterine contraction.

The posterior pituitary is also called the neurohypophysis. It is related to the hypothalamus via the hypothalamo-hypophyseal tract which lies within the hypophyseal stalk. It produces two peptide hormones, vasopressin (ADH, anti-diuretic hormone) and oxytocin, which are structually related.

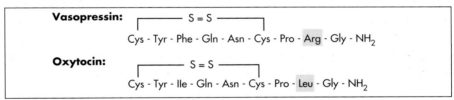

Vasopressin:
```
              ┌──── S = S ────┐
Cys - Tyr - Phe - Gln - Asn - Cys - Pro - Arg - Gly - NH₂
```

Oxytocin:
```
              ┌──── S = S ────┐
Cys - Tyr - Ile - Gln - Asn - Cys - Pro - Leu - Gly - NH₂
```

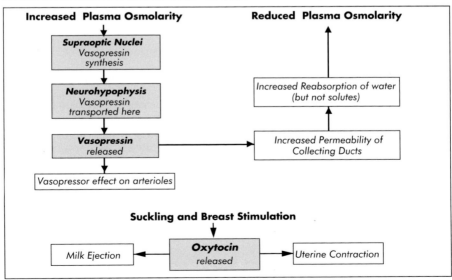

2. WHAT ARE THE FUNCTIONS OF ANTIDIURETIC HORMONE?

⊃ **Classify the different sites of action as a 'framework'.**

1. Antidiuretic hormone (ADH or vasopressin) causes increased distal nephron permeability to water via an action on the aquaporin-2 receptor . This results in greater retrieval of water from the distal nephron and less urine production.
2. Direct vasoconstriction.
   - ▨ Coronary
   - ▨ Splanchnic
   - ▨ Pulmonary
3. Smooth muscle contraction.
4. Stimulation of clotting factor production. This is an endothelial phenomenon of minor significance.

---

3. WHAT ARE THE FUNCTIONS OF THYROID HORMONE?

⊃ **Thyroid hormones have a variety of roles. The important metabolic functions are mediated by intracellular receptors.**

1. Sensitisation of myocardium to catecholamines; by increasing β-receptor synthesis
2. Basal metabolic rate increase (possibly by Na/K-ATPase activity)
3. Reflexes and central nervous system (CNS) enhancement
4. Growth Hormone facilitation
5. CNS development
6. Increased carbohydrate absorption (which increases plasma glucose after meals)
7. Lowering of plasma cholesterol

Mechanism of action:
1. T_3 enters cells and binds nuclear receptors
2. Hormone-receptor complex binds DNA, and increases expression of certain genes
3. Messenger RNAs are formed; these are proteins which alter cellular function

---

4. HOW IS THYROID HORMONE FORMED?

⊃ Thyroid hormone is formed in the thyroid gland from intestinally–absorbed iodine (in ionised form) and tyrosine, which is present as thyroglobulin.

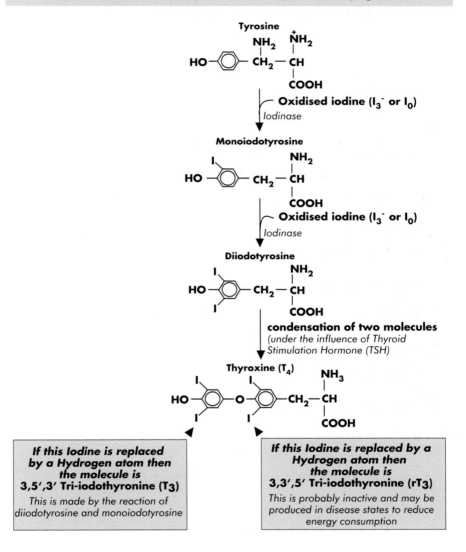

TSH performs three functions:

1. It encourages the uptake of iodine from the gut
2. It converts di-iodothyronine into thyroxine
3. It causes the release of T3 and T4 into the blood

5.   HOW IS BODY TEMPERATURE MAINTAINED?

> ⊃ Humans are homeotherms, with circadian rhythms. Temperature is highest during awake state and at ovulation. Discuss in the order of receptors–comparators–effectors.

Receptors:

These are central and peripheral. The central receptors are the most important and actually regulate body temperature by influencing neural and hormonal changes. Peripheral receptors help by providing information on the how hot or cold the body part is, and so may influence behaviour.

- ▨ Central:
  - Hypothalamus
  - Spinal cord
  - Abdominal viscera
- ▨ Peripheral:
  - Skin
  - Mucous membranes

Comparator:

- ▨ Hypothalamus

Effectors:

- ▨ Neuronal
- ▨ Hormonal; T_4, epinephrine

Mechanisms increasing heat and causing heat preservation:

1. Vasoconstriction and piloerection
2. Behavioural patterns: curl up, seek shelter, increase clothing
3. Shivering, which generates heat but at considerable energy expense
4. Increased activity
5. Non-shivering thermogenesis; this takes place in brown fat, and is observed only in neonates

Mechanisms decreasing heat and allowing for heat dissipation:

1. Vasodilatation
2. Sweating; this is a cholinergic mediated function
3. Hyperventilation. Dogs hyperventilate dead space, eliminating heat, but not ventilating alveoli, which is why they don't pass out while panting
4. Decreased activity

6. CAN YOU DESCRIBE ENDOGENOUS CORTICOSTEROID PRODUCTION?

> ⊃ Use a piece of paper to draw the hypothalamic–pituitary–adrenal cortex axis.

Basal endogenous cortisol production is 25 mg per day. The plasma concentration is subject to a circadian pattern, peaking at about 7 am and the half-life of cortisol is about 90 minutes.

Corticotrophin releasing hormone (CRH) is a 41 amino acid peptide. Both CRH and arginine vasopressin will cause release of adrenocorticotrophic hormone (ACTH) from the anterior lobe of the pituitary. CRH is delivered in the portal system of the pituitary, whereas AVP is present systemically.

ACTH is formed from a precursor molecule, pro-opiomelanocortin. ACTH is blood borne and stimulates production of cortisol from the adrenal cortex. The substrate for cortisol production is cholesterol. Among other steps in the synthesis of cortisol, is a 17 β hydroxylation. This step is inhibited by the induction agent etomidate.

The initial production of corticotrophin releasing hormone from the hypothalamus is stimulated by serotonin and inhibited by norepinephrine. Acetylcholine is implicated in the circadian rhythm and this is abolished by opioid administration. Cortisol itself causes a negative feedback on steroid production at both a hypothalamic and pituitary level.

---

7. WHAT ARE THE FUNCTIONS OF THE PANCREAS?

> ⊃ These should be divided in to endocrine and exocrine.

Endocrine:
- Insulin secretion from β cells
- Glucagon secretion from α cells
- Somatostatin secretion from δ cells

Exocrine (pancreatic juice):
- Trypsin
- Chymotrypsin
- Elastase
- Carboxpeptidases
- Colipase
- α amylase
- Ribonucleases
- Phospholipase-A

These digestive enzymes are secreted as zymogen granules, which are released by exocytosis.

5

QUESTIONS IN GASTROINTESTINAL PHYSIOLOGY

1. DESCRIBE THE ACT OF SWALLOWING?

> ⊃ Simply 'Up–back–shut–shut–swallow'.

Mastication puts a bolus on the dorsum of the tongue.

Styloglossus → Pulls root of tongue up and back.

So: Bolus is pushed up and back against hard palate.

Palatoglossus → Pulls tongue upwards.

So: Bolus is forced into the oropharynx.

Levator } veli palatinii → Elevate soft palate and close off nasopharynx from oropharynx.

Tensor } So: The bolus can't go up the nose.

Stylopharyngeus
Salpingopharyngeus } Elevate the larynx and close the epiglottis.
Palatopharyngeus
and Thyrohyoid

So: Bolus can't enter larynx.

Superior
Middle } Constrictors → Successively contract
Inferior   So: The bolus forced is into the oesophagus.

N.B. 1. Upper fibres of superior constrictor also help to occlude the nasopharynx.
 2. Lower fibres of inferior constrictor form the cricopharyngeus muscle.

2. WHAT IS THE MECHANISM OF VOMITING?

> ⊃ **Clear the route – squeeze – open – vomit.**

1. Deep breath
2. Raise hyoid and larynx to pull crico-oesophageal sphincter open
3. Close glottis
4. Elevation of soft palate to close off nasopharynx
5. Contraction of diaphragm and abdominal muscles, raising intra-abdominal pressure
6. Open gastro-oesophageal sphincter

---

3. HOW IS LIVER BLOOD FLOW REGULATED?

> ⊃ **The liver receives about 40% of cardiac output, 100 ml/100 g tissue/min. It has a dual supply, 500 ml/min from the hepatic artery, which is 95% saturated, and 1000 ml/min from the hepatic portal vein, which is 70% saturated.**

Control is passive and active. Normal O_2 extraction is <50%, if demand increases extraction increases initially.

Active control is intrinsic or extrinsic; intrinsic depends on hepatic artery/hepatic portal vein reciprocity.

Extrinsic control:
- *Sympathetics*: These decrease liver blood flow and liver blood volume; this is a reservoir function.
- *Drugs*: Vasopressin – lowers portal pressure.

---

4. WHAT IS BARRIER PRESSURE?

> ⊃ **Barrier pressure is lower oesophageal sphincter pressure (LOSP) minus intragastric pressure.**

If a pressure transducer were passed from oesophagus into stomach, a pattern would be observed. Initially, thoracic pressure is transmitted across the oesophageal wall, and varies with respiration. After the lower oesophageal sphincter, stomach pressure changes with gastric contractions and diaphragmatic movement.

The significance is that LOSP is reduced by pregnancy, drugs (atropine, suxamethonium) and that intragastric pressure is increased in the fed state. When one encroaches on the other, barrier pressure fails and reflux is possible.

---

5. HOW IS FAT ABSORBED FROM THE GUT?

⊃ Fat is the same as triglyceride; the absorption is a two-stage process.

⊃ Bile salts do two things.

1. They cause emulsification of fat
2. They act to form micelles in order to move the glyceride further down the gut

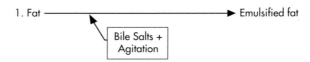

This is by reduction in surface tension of large globules, making small globules, then smaller globules, and finally an emulsion.

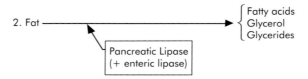

However the glycerides could re-combine with the fatty acids; but bile salts form the glycerides into micelles and move further down the lumen to be absorbed else-where, so that this does not happen.

6. WHAT IS THE COMPOSITION AND FUNCTION OF BILE?

⊃ Bile is produced at 1–2 litres/day and has six main components:

1. Bile salts
2. Cholesterol } these are synthesised in liver, and emulsify fat in the gut.
3. Lecithin
4. Bicarbonate ion: this neutralises gastric acid in the duodenum.
5. Bile pigments
6. Trace metals } these contribute to the elimination of metabolic products.

7. CAN YOU LIST THE FUNCTIONS OF THE LIVER?

1. Production of bile
2. Excretion of bilirubin
3. Storage of glucose as glycogen
4. Formation of Acetoacetic acid from Acetyl CoA as end point of fatty acid metabolism
5. Kupffer cells are part of the reticuloendothelial system, and cleanse portal venous blood
6. Production of plasma proteins
7. Production of clotting factors
8. Formation of urea from ammonia
9. Metabolism of drugs and toxins in two stages/phases
    - ▪ Metabolism: oxidation/hydrolysis/sulphation
    - ▪ Conjugation
10. Blood reservoir
11. Generation of heat

There is a countercurrent mechanism at work. The hepatic sinusoid, which contains hepatic portal venous blood, flows in the opposite direction to the bile canaliculus.

---

8. WHAT IS THE COMPOSITION OF GASTRIC JUICE, AND WHAT STIMULATES ITS PRODUCTION?

Composition:

SUBSTANCE	ORIGIN	CELLULAR SOURE	LOCATION
Acid: HCl: 2 l/day	H+ATPase pump	Parietal cells	Body of stomach
Pepsinogen: ($\rightarrow$ Pepsin)	Protein synthesis	Chief cells	Body and antrum
Mucus	Glycoprotein	Cells at top of gastric glands	Entirety of stom

Production:

PHASE	MEDIATING MECHANISMS	RESULT
Cephalic phase	Parasympathetics, Gastrin	↑HCl
Gastric phase	Long and short neural reflexes, Gastrin	↑HCl
Intestinal phase	Long and short neural reflexes, Secretin, Cholecystokinin	↓HCl

---

9. WHAT ARE THE POTENTIAL PROBLEMS ASSOCIATED WITH DELAYED GASTRIC EMPTYING AND WHAT ARE THE CAUSES ?

⊃ **The problems are aspiration of stomach contents, alteration in the absorption characteristics of oral drugs, and nausea and vomiting. ITU patients typically have delayed gastric emptying.**

Causes:

1. **Physiological**
   - Food and increased osmotic load (jejunal receptors delay emptying to allow controlled release)
   - Posture (especially in neonates)
   - Anxiety ('state' more important than 'trait')
   - Age (some delay in liquid emptying in the elderly)

3. **Pharmacological**
   - Opioids including partial opiate agonists such as meptazinol, nalbuphine, buprenorphine and nefopam
     - Epidural opioids
   - Anticholinergics
     - Atropine
     - Tricyclic antidepressants
     - Ganglion blockers
   - Aluminium and Magnesium hydroxides
   - Sympathomimetic drugs
     - Salbutamol
     - Isoprenaline
     - Dopamine
   - Alcohol

2. **Pathological**
   - GI obstruction
   - Acute gastroparesis
     - Migraine
     - Acute gastro-enteritis
     - Hypercalcaemia
     - Electrolyte imbalance
     - Diabetes Mellitus
     - Raised intracranial pressure
   - Muscular disorders
   - Anorexia nervosa
   - Acute renal failure
   - Crohn's disease
   - Myxoedema

4. **Other Factors**
   - Pregnancy; no consistent effect
   - Obesity: Solid emptying is **increased**, but liquid emptying is **normal**; the residual volume of gastric secretions is **higher**.

6

QUESTIONS ON RENAL PHYSIOLOGY

1. CAN YOU DESCRIBE THE COUNTERCURRENT MECHANISM OF THE KIDNEY?

> ⟳ A countercurrent fluid mechanism is one in which fluid flows through a long U–tube with the two limbs of the U tube lying in close proximity so that exchange of constituents may take place between the two arms.

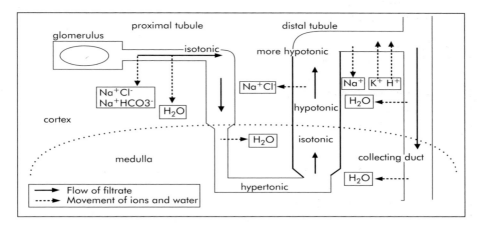

In the loop of Henle, osmolality at the tip is 1200 mosm/l in the lumen and in the interstitium.

The Key is that the ascending limb (the thick portion, which is known as the diluting segment) is impervious to Na^+ and Cl^- ions and has a powerful Na^+ pump moving Na^+ and Cl^- ions into the interstitium. This maintains the composition of the interstitium of the renal medulla at high osmolality.

The purpose is that extremely dilute urine is generated at the distal tubule, which then passes through the highly concentrated milieu of the medulla. The barrier between the two is formed by the collecting duct, whose normally impervious wall can be made permeable to water by the action of ADH. The osmolality of the urine can be adjusted by varying the permeability of the collecting duct to water.

---

2. WHAT ARE THE PRESSURES WITHIN THE GLOMERULUS?

> ⊃ Hydrostatic pressure is higher in glomerular capillary beds than in other organs.

High capillary pressure is maintained by balance between afferent (precapillary) and efferent (postcapillary) arterioles. Hydrostatic pressure is normally maintained at about 90 mmHg.

Against this is:

- 25 mmHg plasma oncotic pressure
- 15 mmHg Bowman's capsule hydrostatic pressure

Therefore filtration pressure is about 50 mmHg. This is consistent with:

- The filtration function of the kidney
- Oliguria being an early feature as arterial pressure falls

3. WHAT HAPPENS TO THE CONCENTRATION OF SODIUM, GLUCOSE AND INULIN AS THE FILTRATE PASSES DOWN THE PROXIMAL CONVOLUTED TUBULE?

> ⊃ $^2/_3$ of water reabsorption takes place in the proximal convoluted tubule (PCT).

- Inulin is filtered but not reabsorbed, therefore its concentration rises
- Glucose concentration is zero
- Sodium concentration is unchanged; water is reabsorbed with sodium

4. HOW IS GLOMERULAR FILTRATION RATE CONTROLLED?

> ⊃ Glomerular filtration is the volume of fluid filtered from glomerular capillaries into Bowman's capsule per unit time. It is 180 l/day (120 ml/min) in the adult.

Glomerular filtration rate (GFR) is proportional to glomerular capillary pressure. This in turn depends on:

1. Local autoregulation, mediated by renal sympathetic nerves. Increased sympathetic activity causes increased afferent vasoconstriction, and decreased glomerular pressure.
2. Mean arterial pressure.

5. HOW DOES THE KIDNEY EXCRETE H⁺ ION?

> ⊃ **This concerns carbonic anhydrase.**

Control of pH is proportional to $\left|\begin{array}{l} H^+ \text{ elimination} \\ HCO_3\text{- reabsorption} \end{array}\right.$

- ▒ The intracellular buffers are phosphates and proteins (especially Hb)
- ▒ The extracellular buffer is principally bicarbonate (and some proteins)
- ▒ The urinary buffers are HPO_4^{2-} and NH_3, and a very little bicarbonate

A diagram may provide an opportunity to explain and for further discussion: start by drawing the renal cell, and the CO_2 and H_2O within it:

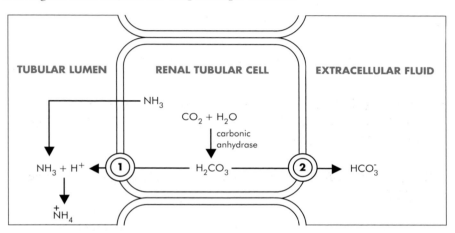

The separate parts of the tubular system are driven by two distinct processes as the transport at 1 and 2 above differ:

A. Early tubular segments (proximal tubule, thick segment of the ascending limb of the loop of Henle and distal tubule):

- ▒ **At 1:** H^+ is secreted by Na^+/H^+ countertransport (a process driven by the lower intracellular concentration of sodium).
- ▒ **At 2:** The sodium is then transported out of the cell to the extracellular space by Na^+/K^+-ATPase, and HCO_3- passes out to balance the electrical effect of the extra sodium pumped out.

B. Late tubular segments (late distal tubules then on through the remainder of the system to the renal pelvis):

- ▒ **At 1:** H^+ is secreted by primary active transport utilising a specific transport protein H^+-transporting ATPase.
- ▒ **At 2:** The HCO_3- is exchanged for a chloride ion that passes out to the tubule with the hydrogen ion and so ensures electrical neutrality.

6. HOW IS GLUCOSE HANDLED BY THE KIDNEY?

> ⊃ Differentiate between the normal and disease states. Normally there is
> no glucose in the urine.

Normally almost all filtered glucose is reabsorbed (a negligble amount is excreted). Most glucose reabsorption occurs in the proximal tubule but the distal nephron is also capable of glucose absorption. the amount of glucose filtered is directly proportional to the plasma glucose concentration. Provided the plasma glucose concentration remains below 11 mmol/l there is no excretion of glucose into the urine. Above this however nephrons with a lower capacity for glucose reabsorption (and remember that the capacity does vary between nephrons) will exceed their capacity leading to the appearance of glucose in theurine. this is obviously seen in diabetic states. At a plasma glucose concentration of 22 mmol/l no nephrons can absorb their filtered load. Any solute has a maximum tubular transport rate – The T_m. These values vary between nephrons.

7. WHAT IS RPF? HOW IS IT MEASURED?

> ⊃ RPF is renal plasma flow.

Renal plasma flow describes the amount of plasma passing through the renal circulation in one minute. The normal value is 625 ml/min in the adult. Since the kidney filters plasma, RPF will equate to the amount of a substance excreted per unit time divided by the renal A-V difference (this assumes no entry into red cells). Although any substance could be used if; it can be measured in renal arterial and venous plasma, it is not metabolised, stored nor affects renal blood flow, in practice para-amino hippuric acid (PAH) is used.

To convert RPF to renal blood flow (1200 ml/min) use the formula:

$$RBF = RPF \times \frac{1}{1 - Haematocrit}$$

7

QUESTIONS IN METABOLIC PHYSIOLOGY AND BIOCHEMISTRY

1. WHAT IS THE DIFFERENCE BETWEEN OSMOLALITY AND OSMOLARITY?

Concentration:
MolaRity is the number of moles per litRe of solution.

MolaLity is the number of moles per kiLogram of solvent.

Osmotic pressure:
- Osmolarity expresses mmol *per litre* of solution
- Oxmolality expresses mmol *per kilogram* of solvent

Measurement:
1. Depression of freezing point: This is the osmotic effect exerted by sum of all dissolved molecules and ions across a membrane permeable only to water.
2. Calculated:
   Total $= 2\,[Na^+ + K^+] + [urea] + [glucose]$

> ⊃ All units are mmol/l.
> The factor of 2 for Na^+ and K^+ allows for equal quantities of associated anions and assumes complete ionisation.
> Normal serum osmolarity is 290 mmol/l.

Significance:
1. Direct measurement by depression of freezing point indicates osmolality.
2. Calculation indicates osmolarity.
3. Urine contains no protein, whereas plasma contains about 70 g/l of protein. This means that the total volume (water + protein) is about 6% greater than that of the solvent (the water alone). Measured osmolality will be greater than calculated osmolarity.
4. In reality, there is little difference between osmolarity and osmolality other than when there is extreme hyperlipidaemia or hyperproteinaemia.
5. Comparison of plasma and urine must be done in terms of osmolality of both, in other words, by direct measurement.
6. Total osmotic pressure of plasma is 7 atmospheres.

2. WHAT ARE THE PHYSIOLOGICAL ACTIONS OF INSULIN?

⊃ **Insulin is the main anabolic hormone, and its action is opposed by all stress hormones.**

1. Activation of glucose uptake
2. Concurrent uptake of [K^+]
3. Glycogen synthesis
4. Increased lipogenesis
5. Inhibition of gluconeogenesis
6. Inhibition of glycogenolysis
7. Inhibition of ketogenesis
8. Inhibition of lipolysis
9. Enhancement of protein synthesis from amino acids

---

3. WHERE IS IRON PRESENT IN THE BODY, AND HOW IS IT ABSORBED?

⊃ **Iron is present in the body as follows:**

- 70% in haemoglobin, Hb
- 25% in ferritin
- 5% myoglobin

The functions are:
1. In globin, within haemoglobin, as O_2 binding site for transport.
2. In globin, within myoglobin, as O_2 binding site for collection and storage.

Only 10% of total iron ingested is absorbed. Active transport transfers iron from the gut to ferritin within the intestinal cells and then to the liver. Ferritin effectively regulates the uptake of iron; the more body iron, the more intestinal iron, and the less iron absorbed.

- Ferritin (mostly hepatic) is a storage protein iron complex
- Transferrin is a plasma protein (transport)

Most of the intestinal cell ferritin is lost when the cell reaches the top of the villus and drops off.

Conclusion
The affinity of ferritin for iron is reduced when iron is scarce – by an unknown mechanism – allowing more iron to enter circulation and bind transferrin.

---

4. WHAT IS NORMAL EXTRA CELLULAR FLUID VOLUME AND HOW IS IT MEASURED?

⊃ **Extracellular fluid (ECF) is 20% of body weight. ECF is one third of total body water — 14 l.**

ECF is distributed:
- Intravascularly: 4 l
- Interstitially: 10 l

Measurement is difficult because few substances mix readily. Lymph cannot be measured separately. Substances cross the blood brain barrier slowly and don't equilibrate well.

Measurement is also difficult because of the existence of transcellular fluids:

- Glandular secretions
- CSF
- Aqueous humour

The method commonly described is of radioactive Inulin, which has a molecular weight of 5200; using a 14C substitution and dilution technique. (Inulin is also used in measurement of GFR) Cl⁻ and Br⁻ labelling doesn't work because these molecules are intracellular.

$$\text{Volume} = \frac{\text{quantity injected}}{\text{concentration observed}}$$

5. WHAT IS THE ANION GAP?

⊃ **The anion gap has been used to calculate plasma acidity**
$= ([Na^+]+[K^+]) - ([Cl^-]+[HCO_3^-])$; normal = 10–15 mmol/l.

The anion gap is increased by:
- Increased serum lactate – but lactate can be directly measured now, so the anion gap has become a less frequently used measurement
- Ketoacidosis
- Increased foreign anions, salicylates for example
- Hypocalcaemia
- Hypokalaemia
- Hypomagnesaemia

The anion gap is decreased by:
- Hypoalbuminaemia
- Increased plasma cations

6. HOW IS BODY WATER DISTRIBUTED?

> ⊃ Body water is 60% of body weight.

TOTAL 42 l – Intracellular 24 l
             – Extracellular   Plasma 4 l
                                Interstitial 10 l

                                Bone 4 l

In:			Out:		
Fluid	2500		Urine	1500
Food	750		Skin	600
Metabolic	350		Resp	400
	2600		Stool	100
				2600

Total Secretions: (most of which are reabsorbed)
Saliva   1500
Gastric   2500
Bile   1000
Pancreas   700
Small gut   3000
             ≈ 9000 ml/day; implications for fistulae are obvious.

7. WHAT ARE THE FUNCTIONS OF CALCIUM IN THE BODY?

> ⊃ Apart from the 99% of the total which is in bone, calcium is a
> predominantly extracellular ion; when it is present in the intracellular
> compartment, it exerts profound effects and is a component of many
> second–messenger systems.

1. Bone salt: Ca^{2+}: PO_4^{2-} 2: 1, as $Ca_{10}(PO_4)_6(OH)_2$
2. Glycogen breakdown requires transient Ca^{2+} release to activate phosphorylase kinase.
3. Muscle contraction: Depolarisation causes Ca^{2+} release from sarcoplasmic reticulum, affecting the TpC component of troponin, which in turn elicits a tropomyosin-actin conformational change; this causes a contraction.
4. Release of acetylcholine depends on presence of Ca^{2+} in the extracellular fluid.
5. Calcium is a neurotransmitter in the generation of the visual impulse, by closure of Na^+ gates.
6. Clotting: Calcium is factor IV in the intrinsic and extrinsic pathways.
7. Vasoconstriction: Calcium is the biochemical antagonist of K^+.
8. The plateau of the cardiac action potential depends on slow Ca^{2+} channel activity.
9. It is a positive inotrope.

8. WHICH AMINO ACIDS ARE ESSENTIAL?

> ⊃ As a mnemonic "<u>Little</u> <u>most</u> – <u>valuable</u> – <u>player</u>"

Leucine
Isoleucine
Threonine
Tryptophan
Lysine
Methionine
Valine
Phenylalanine; hence tyrosine is not essential unless phenylalanine is absent.

Bone + Teeth

9. HOW IS PHOSPHATE PRESENT IN THE BODY? - *soft Skeleton*

1. Phosphate is present in association with calcium, as the anion.
2. It is present as a buffer in glomerular filtrate to allow excretion of H^+ and generation of HCO_3^-.
3. It is a component of high-energy phosphate bonds; adenosine monophosphate, (AMP), adenosine diphosphate (ADP), and adenosine triphosphate (ATP). Insulin facilitates cellular PO_4^- uptake.

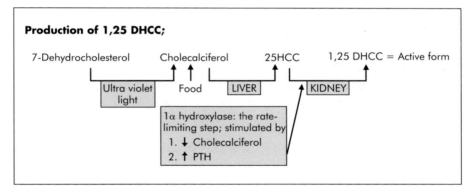

Production of 1,25 DHCC;

Calcitonin opposes these actions.

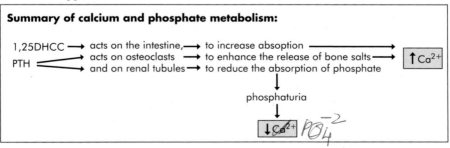

Summary of calcium and phosphate metabolism:

---

10. CAN YOU COMPARE THE NERNST AND GOLDMAN EQUATIONS?

> ⊃ Nernst describes the electric potential necessary to balance a given ionic concentration gradient across a membrane so that the net passive flux of the ion is zero.

This is analogous to osmotic pressure – the effort required to stop movement.

$$E \quad = \quad \frac{RT}{zF} \quad \log_e \quad \frac{[C_o]}{[C_I]}$$

E $\quad = \quad$ equilibrium potential of the ion in question

$C_o, C_i \quad = \quad$ extra and intracellular concentrations

z $\quad = \quad$ valance of ion in question

R $\quad = \quad$ gas constant $\quad$ 8314.9 J/kg.mol.K

T $\quad = \quad$ absolute temp in Kelvin

F $\quad = \quad$ Faraday constant = quantity of electricity in 1 mole elections

$\quad = \quad$ 96,484 6 c/mol

For Potassium:

$$E \quad = \quad \frac{8314 \times 310}{1 \times 96,484} \quad \times \quad \log_e \quad \frac{4}{140}$$

$$E \quad = \quad 26.7 \quad \times \quad \log_e \quad 0.028$$

So, the larger the extracellular $[K^+]$, the larger the potential difference.

> ⊃ Goldman takes account of Na, Cl and other ions.

$$V_m \quad = \quad \frac{RT}{F} \log_e \frac{P_K \times K_o + P_{Na} \times Na_o + P_{Cl} \times Cl_i}{P_K \times K_i + P_{Na} \times Na_i + P_{Cl} \times Cl_o}$$

P = membrane permeabilities – which can alter, so turning the Goldman equation into the Nernst equation for that particular ion.

11. HOW ARE CYTOKINES IMPLICATED IN THE DEVELOPMENT OF SEPSIS?

Cytokines are low molecular weight proteins that act as local factors in inflammatory and immune responses. They have a short half-life but are extremely potent, interacting with receptors on membrane surfaces. The actions of cytokines are exceedingly complex and there is considerable overlapping of actions, as well as positive feedback and amplification (as with the complement cascade). They are believed to be the final pathway for the organ and cell damage that is the result of sepsis. The important cytokines are interleukin-1 (IL-1), interleukin-6 (IL-6) and tumour necrosis factor (TNF), and their actions are summarised in the following table:

CYTOKINE	SOURCE	ACTIVATING FACTORS	EFFECTS
IL-1	Vascular endothelium Vascular smooth muscle Macrophages	Tissue injury Exotoxin Endotoxin TNF Complement	Reduced systematic vascular resistance Fever Amplification of TNF effects
IL-6	Vascular endothelium	TNF C5a complement factor	Synthesis of acute phase proteins Fever
TNF	Vascular endothelium Vascular smooth muscle Macrophage	Tissue injury Exotoxin Endotoxin TNF Complement	Reduce systemic vascular resistance by enhanced vasodilation and reduced vasoconstriction Lactic acidosis Hypoglycaemia Expression of adhesion molecules on vascular endothelium Margination and adherence of neutrophils, monocytes and lymphocytes Activation of neutrophils Increased vascular permeability Self-amplification Release of IL-1 and IL-6 Release of catecholamines, glucagon, cortisol, PAF, arachidonic acid derivatives, interferons

12. DEFINE BASAL METABOLIC RATE AND FACTORS AFFECTING THE METABOLIC RATE

⊃ Basal metabolic rate is energy necessary to maintain essential processes such as beating of the heart, respiration and thermoregulation. It is determined at rest in a room of thermoneutral temperature (28 degrees Celsius), 12 to 14 hours after the last meal.

It is expressed as $kJ/m^2/hour$.

An average person has a basal metabolic rate of 2000 kcal/day.

Factors affecting the basal metabolic rate are:

- Muscle exertion
- Recent ingestion of food
- Temperature of environment
- Height, weight, surface area, age and gender of subject
- Emotional state
- Body temperature
- Circulating levels of thyroxine and cathecholamines

⊃ How would you measure the basal metabolic rate?

Oxygen consumption is measured using a Benedict spirometer filled with oxygen that has been modified to include a carbon dioxide absorber. The spirometer bell is connected to a pen that marks the rotating drum as the bell moves up and down. The slope of the line is proportional to the amount of oxygen consumed. This amount (in millilitres) per unit time is corrected to standard temperature and pressure and multiplied by 4.82 kcal/l to convert to energy used.

---

13. WHAT MARKERS OF NUTRITIONAL STATE DO YOU KNOW?

- Mid arm circumference triceps skin fold thickness
- Mid thigh circumference
- Plasma proteins example albumin, transferring
- Immune function (e.g. lymphocyte count)

---

14. WHAT IS THE RESPONSE TO STARVATION?

First 2 days: Glycogenolysis occurs

Increased insulin production inhibits protein breakdown in muscle therefore giving a protein sparing effect.

First week: Gluconeogenesis occurs

Muscle protein is mobilised as alanine (preferred substrate for hepatic gluconeogenesis) or glutamine (preferred substrate for renal gluconeogenesis).

Second week: Ketoadaptation occurs as gluconeogenesis decreases

Fats are converted to ketoacids and when fat stores are depleted, protein catabolism increases and death follows.

⊃ **What are the endocrine changes associated with starvation?**

- **Insulin** decreases secondary to decline in body glucose
- **Glucagon** increases in the first three to four days
- **Cathecolamines** increase in the first 24 hours and increase the basal metabolic rate: in the long term there is decreased sympathetic nervous system activity
- **Growth hormone** is increased until day 10 and is associated with gluconeogenesis
- **Cortisol** is elevated in prolonged starvation
- **Tetraiodotyrosine** (T_4) increased in first three days then returns to normal by day 10

_____

PHARMACOLOGY

1

QUESTIONS ON ANAESTHETIC DRUGS

1. WHAT ARE THE TOXIC EFFECTS OF LOCAL ANAESTHETICS?

> ⊃ These can be due to overdose, as part of the therapeutic effect, or due
> to the addition of a vasoconstrictor or other additive; anaphylaxis
> although possible is very rare.

Due to overdose:
  a. Central nervous system: Esters (procaine and cocaine) cause central nervous
      system depression, while amides cause central nervous system depression
      then fits, in other words, there is a biphasic response
  b. Cardiovascular system: Hypotension and brady-arrhythmias
  c. The 'total spinal' with cardiovascular collapse and apnoea

As part of therapeutic effect:
  a. Respiratory depression in intercostal block
  b. Autonomic blockade (spinals)

Vasoconstrictor addition:
  a. Digital extremities and the penis are vulnerable to unwanted
      vasoconstriction and there is a possibility of gangrene ·
  b. Vasopressors may cause a hypertensive crisis if used where psychiatric drugs
      such as uptake-1 inhibitors are present

Specific effects:
  Type I hypersensitivity (Ester group, seen with cocaine)

Safe doses: See Table below

MAXIMUM RECOMMENDED DOSES (AND THEIR MG/KG EQUIVALENTS)				
	Adult dose (mg)		mg/kg equivalent	
	Plain	With epinephrine	Plain	With epinephrine
Ester				
Cocaine	100	*	1.5	*
Amide				
Bupivacaine	150	150	2	2
Lidocaine	200	500	3	7
Prilocaine	400	600 (felypressin)	6	8.5
Ropivacaine**	250	N/A	3.5	N/A
*Unnecessary and contraindicated				
**150 mg (2 mg/kg) for epidural Caesarean section				

---

2.   COMPARE BUPIVACAINE AND LIDOCAINE.

⊃ They are both are amide local anaesthetics but have different properties in terms of potency, duration of action and physical characteristics.

	BUPIVACAINE	LIDOCAINE
Potency	4	1
Duration	4	1
Safe max. dose (mg/kg)	2	3
Pka	8.1	7.7
Partition coefficient	28	3
Protein bound	95%	64%

---

3.   CAN YOU COMPARE CENTRAL NERVOUS SYSTEM TOXICITY OF AMIDE AND ESTER LOCAL ANAESTHETICS?

⊃ Procaine is an ester, as is amethocaine and cocaine; lidocaine and most others are amides.

The signs of local anaesthetic toxicity in the nervous system are alterations of conscious level and circumoral tingling. Amides cause initial central nervous system depression, which is then followed by convulsions. Ester local anaesthetics produce no biphasic pattern, just central nervous system depression. Lidocaine toxicity can be related to the concentration in the plasma.

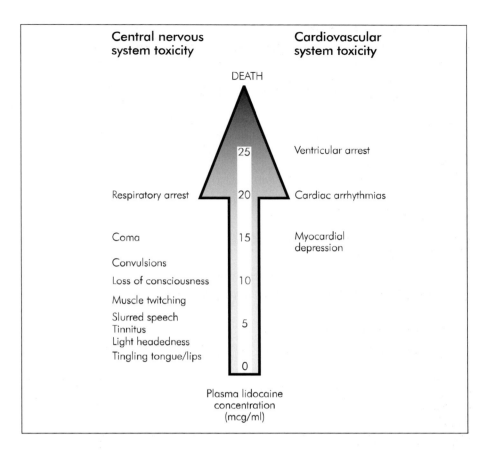

Central nervous system toxicity — Cardiovascular system toxicity

DEATH

CNS	Plasma lidocaine concentration (mcg/ml)	CVS
	25	Ventricular arrest
Respiratory arrest	20	Cardiac arrhythmias
Coma	15	Myocardial depression
Convulsions		
Loss of consciousness	10	
Muscle twitching		
Slurred speech	5	
Tinnitus		
Light headedness		
Tingling tongue/lips		
	0	

Plasma lidocaine concentration (mcg/ml)

4.   WHAT IS MAC?

➲ **Minimum alveolar concentration (MAC) of inhalational anaesthetic agent at sea level, in 100% oxygen, at which 50% of unpremedicated experimental animals will fail to respond to a standard midline incision. This is MAC 50; if considering the concentration which will achieve absence of movement in 90% of patients, then this will be MAC 90. The accepted standard is MAC 50.**

The term minimum is used because it is a threshold level; and it is described as alveolar because it applies at equilibrium.

5. WHAT FACTORS MODIFY MINIMUM ALVEOLAR CONCENTRATION (MAC)?

MAC is reduced by:

1. Age (by 10% per decade)
2. Premedication
3. Opioids
4. Hypovolaemia
5. Reduced temperature
6. Other drugs: for example, clonidine, dexmedetomidine
7. Disease: hypothyroidism

6. WHAT IS IN THE THIOPENTONE AMPOULE?

> ⊃ Ignorance of this will go down very badly. This topic is often linked with pKa because alkalising a weak acid such as thiopentone increases its water solubility.

The drug is prepared as a sodium salt. It is a 2.5% powder of 5 Ethyl, 5′ methylbutyl thiobarbituric acid; pH is 10.5. All salts of weak acids are alkaline in solution. The preparation also contains 6 parts per 100 of Na_2CO_3 which produces OH^- ions in solution thus preventing precipitation of free acid form of drug and aiding water solubility. The powder is presented in an atmosphere of nitrogen in order to prevent oxidation in the bottle.

7. WHAT FACTORS MODIFY THIOPENTONE DOSAGE?

> ⊃ "Modify" implies both enhancement and reduction of effects.

An enhanced effect is seen in:
- The elderly
- Malnutrition (because of reduced protein binding)
- The debilitated
- Hypovolaemia
- Premedicated patients
- Hyperventilation, which is also a phenomenon of displacement from protein binding

Reduced effects are seen in:
- Enzyme induction (Hepatic P_{450} mixed function oxidase)
- Chronic alcohol abuse – mainly a cellular tolerance

8. WHAT IS THE SIGNIFICANCE OF THE OIL–GAS PARTITION COEFFICIENT?

⊃ It is an index of potency and is inversely related to MAC. This lends itself to a diagram.

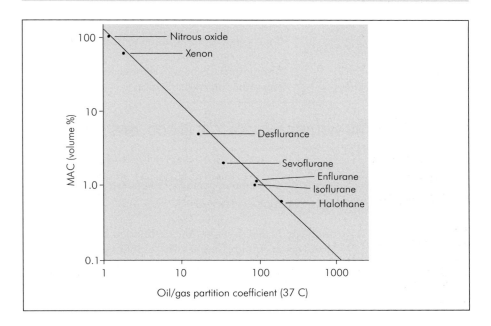

This relationship supports the Meyer-Overton hypothesis of the mechanism of action of anaesthetics, namely that the action is related to the lipid solubility of the agent and takes place at the level of the central nervous system cell membrane. If the Meyer-Overton hypothesis were correct, then the product of MAC and the oil: gas partition coefficient would be a single constant. However the MAC-O: G product produced by the newer agents (sevoflurane, desflurane and isoflurane) is approximately 100 and that of the older agents (e.g. enflurane and halothane) is approximately 200, perhaps suggesting two different sites of action or mechanisms.

The multi-site expansion hypothesis suggests that the sites at which anaesthetics operate have finite size and limited occupancy. When considering volatile agents, MAC is additive, but although opioids reduce MAC they do not do so in a predictable, additive fashion, which suggests that they are not having the effect at the same site as the anaesthetic agent. There is also evidence that anaesthetic agents work at synaptic level, possibly at the thalamic level of the central nervous system. As knowledge of the mechanism of action of anaesthetic drugs slowly emerges it appears that an effect on the cell membrane will be the most likely site of effect.

9. HOW IS NITROUS OXIDE MANUFACTERED?

> ⊃ By heating Ammonium Nitrate to 245°C

$$NH_4NO_3 \rightarrow N_2O + 2H_2O$$

The end product may contain impurities:

▓ Ammonia
▓ Nitric Acid } On cooling these combine to form NH_4NO_3
▓ Nitrogen
▓ Nitric oxide (NO) | Aluminium dryers will remove these; N_2
▓ Nitrogen dioxide (NO_2) | evaporates off by distillation

10. WHAT IS THE SIGNIFICANCE OF THE BLOOD: GAS PARTITION COEFFICIENT?

> ⊃ There has always been confusion among candidates between the oil: gas, and the blood: gas, partition coefficients.

The blood: gas (B:G) partition coefficient describes the partition of a volatile anaesthetic agent between blood and gas at equilibrium. Poorly soluble agents have a low B:G coefficient, whereas highly soluble agents will have a high coefficient. Desflurane (insoluble) has a B:G coefficient around 0.4, whereas diethyl ether (soluble) has a B:G coefficient of 12.

There is a paradox in the relationship between B:G solubility and rapidity of action. A highly soluble agent will enter the blood avidly, but exert a low partial pressure. The effects on the central nervous system are related to the partial pressure of the agent, not to the absolute amount present, so a soluble agent will have a slow onset of action. A poorly soluble agent by contrast will exert a rapid effect. Thus cyclopropane was a very effective agent for the gaseous induction of anaesthesia, although desflurane, which has a similar B:G coefficient, is limited in its effectiveness for gaseous induction by the irritation it causes in the respiratory tract. Speed of onset also relates to speed of emergence, and desflurane is associated with a rapid recovery whereas methoxyflurane has a very slow pattern of recovery. Methoxyflurane is no longer used in human practice because of concerns about nephrotoxicity, however it remains a useful agent in veterinary practice because of the one property that made it popular in human practice; it is a potent analgesic.

11. WHAT IS THE NATURE OF ENTONOX?

- $N_2O : O_2$, 50 : 50
- Stored at 137 Bar in cylinder sizes G (3200 l) and J (6400 l)
- Provided in a blue cylinder, with blue and white quartered shoulders
- Separates at $-7°$ which is the 'pseudo-critical' temperature: the liquid contains N_2O with very little O_2 dissolved in it
- Filling ratio 0.75

The existence of Entonox relies on the Poynting effect. The mixed gases do not behave as might be predicted from the characteristics of their components, but rather the two gases appear to dissolve into one another. The mixture is less likely to separate into two phases, under the influence of pressure, than N_2O alone. Thus the mixture is able to remain gaseous at higher pressures and at lower temperatures than N_2O.

---

12. WHAT CAUSES HALOTHANE HEPATITIS?

> ⊃ Halothane is not a classic toxin, because it does not meet the three criteria for a toxin.

1. Observed dose-effect relationship
2. Validity in different animal species
3. Recognised mode of action

Halothane undergoes oxidative and reductive metabolism to produce trifluroacetic acid, chloride, bromide and fluoride. There are two degrees of hepatic damage observed:

1. Reversible damage, associated with mild elevation in hepatic transaminases; this may be sub-clinical.
2. Fulminant necrosis, which is associated with an antibody-antigen reaction. Halothane behaves as a hapten, binding covalently with hepatic proteins, inducing formation of antibodies. This is supposed to be associated with serial and repeated anaesthetics with halothane, and is seen at an incidence of between 1: 82,000 and 1: 200,000 in children, although the incidence of unexplained jaundice in adults following halothane anaesthesia is higher, at between 1: 2,500 and 1: 36,000. The diagnosis of halothane-induced liver damage can only be made after exclusion of all other causes of liver damage.

Although UK usage of halothane is now minimal, it is still extensively used globally especially in third world environments.

---

13. WHAT ARE THE DEGRADATION PRODUCTS OF SEVOFLURANE?

> ⊃ Sevoflurane has been widely used in Japan for several years and is now
> well established in clinical practice in the UK. Early on there were fears
> about degradation products and possible toxicity.

Sevoflurane is absorbed and degraded by carbon dioxide absorbers. At temperatures of 65°C five breakdown products are formed (Compounds A to E). In the lower temperatures encountered clinically sevoflurane only produces Compound A $(CH_2F-O-C(CF_3)=CF_2)$ and a lesser amount of Compound B $(CHF_2-O-CH(CF_2-O-CH_3)-CF_3)$. The concentrations are higher with baralyme than soda lime because baralyme attains a higher temperature and the breakdown is temperature dependent. The concentrations of Compounds A and B are substantially lower than the toxicity threshold in animal studies. Possible toxicity effects are renal, hepatic and brain. A new zeolite coated soda lime may absorb these compounds

14. WHAT IS THE SECOND GAS EFFECT?

> ⊃ This is to do with the much greater solubility of N_2O than N_2 in the
> blood, and the influence of this on P_AO_2 and the alveolar concentration
> of a volatile anaesthetic agent.

The concentration effect is the effect of rapid extraction from the alveolus of a gas introduced at high concentration (such as nitrous oxide). Because the initial uptake of the nitrous oxide from the alveolus is high, the alveolar partial pressures of other simultaneously administered gases (such as volatile anaesthetic agents) will be increased. The second gas effect is effectively a consequence of this, as the F_A/F_I (alveolar fraction to inspired fraction) ratio of the concurrently-administered volatile agent will equilibrate faster than it would in the absence of the nitrous oxide. This means that induction of anaesthesia will be more rapid.

The second gas effect has another consequence. In addition to accelerating induction, the effect may retard recovery by causing "diffusion hypoxia". During emergence from anaesthesia, when air is replacing anaesthetic gas, the nitrous oxide will diffuse from the blood to the alveolus faster than it is replaced in the blood by nitrogen from room air, because of the difference in their solubilities. The ratio of the solubility of nitrogen to nitrous oxide is 1: 35. Therefore the alveolar concentration of nitrous oxide rises, and if the inspired gas is room air, then the partial pressure of oxygen in the alveolus will be reduced below that of room air by the nitrous oxide entering the alveolus faster than the nitrogen is leaving the alveolus. This is one of the reasons why oxygen is routinely administered to patients emerging from anaesthesia.

15. WHAT WOULD BE THE IDEAL VOLATILE ANAESTHETIC AGENT?

Physical:
- Stable in light, heat, metal, soda lime
- No preservatives
- Long shelf life
- Not flammable or explosive
- Non-irritant
- Atmospherically friendly
- Cheap

Pharmacokinetic:
- High oil: gas coefficient, low minimum alveolar concentration (MAC)
- Low blood: gas coefficient, fast effects
- Not metabolised

Pharmacodynamic:
- Non-toxic, even in chronic, low dose
- Absence of, or at least predictable, cardiovascular and respiratory effects
- Analgesic
- Readily reversible anaesthetic effects
- Not epileptogenic
- No interactions
- No effects on the gravid uterus

	MW Daltons	BP at 1 Atm °C	SVP at 20°C kPa	MAC % v/v	blood/ gas	oil/ water	water/ gas	brain/ gas	oil/ gas	brain/ blood
Units										
Desflurane	168	22.8	88.5	6.35	0.42	N/A	N/A	0.54	19	1.3
Enflurane	184.5	56.5	22.9	1.68	1.9	120	0.78	2.6	98	96
Halothane	197	50.2	32.5	0.75	2.3	220	0.8	4.8	224	1.9
Isoflurane	184.5	48.5	31.9	1.15	1.43	174	0.62	21	91	1.6
Sevoflurane	200	58.6	21.3	2.00	0.69	N/A	N/A	1.1	53	1.7
Nitrous oxide	44	-88	5300	105	0.47	3.2	0.44		1.4	
Cyclopropane	42	-33	640	9.2	0.45	34.4	0.2		11.5	
Diethyl ether	74	35	7.8	1.9	12.1	3.2	13		65	
Trichlorethylene	131	87	1.1	0.17	9.15	400	1.7		960	
*Ethyl chloride	64.5	13	132							

* Although no longer used as a volatile agent by inhalation, ethyl chloride remains in practice as a cutaneous analgesic when applied as a spray. It is included here out of completeness.

16. DRAW THE RELATIONSHIP OF INSPIRED CONCENTRATION AGAINST THE ALVEOLAR CONCENTRATION FOR A VOLATILE ANAESTHETIC AGENT.

⊃ **This relates to the blood: gas partition coefficient.**

Poorly soluble volatile agents have a small blood: gas partition coefficient, so alveolar concentration rises rapidly towards inspired concentration, a large gradient exists and onset of anaesthesia is rapid.

N_2O	0.5
Halothane	2.3
Enflurane	1.8
Isoflurane	1.4
Sevoflurane	0.6
Desflurane	0.4 – fastest of all

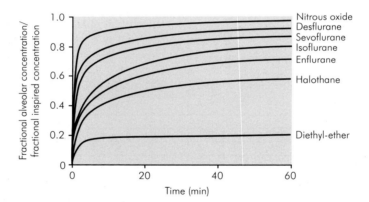

The F_A/F_I ratio rises faster (and therefore induction is faster) in **low** cardiac output and **high** minute ventilation.

17. WHY DOES ALFENTANIL START TO WORK SO MUCH FASTER THAN FENTANYL, AND WHY IS ITS DURATION OF ACTION SO MUCH SHORTER?

⊃ This concerns the pharmacokinetic differences between the two drugs. The relevant data is shown in the following tables:

Drug	Distribution $t_{1/2}$ (min)	Terminal $t_{1/2}$ (min)	Initial volume of distribution (l/kg)	Volume of distribution (l/kg)	Clearance (ml/min)
Fentanyl	13	190	0.85	4.0	1500
Alfentanil	11.6	100	0.16	0.53	240

Drug	Plasma protein binding (% bound)	pKa	% Ionised at pH 7.4
Fentanyl	83	8.4	91
Alfentanil	90	6.5	11

It can be seen that the terminal half-life of alfentanil is half that of fentanyl, but that the clearance of alfentanil is much smaller. Therefore the shorter terminal half-life is due to the smaller volume of distribution of alfentanil – fentanyl is highly lipid soluble and extensively taken up by fat and muscle (this is the main reason for its short duration of action when compared with morphine which has a similar terminal half-life).

As alfentanil is poorly lipid soluble it has a much smaller initial volume of distribution and as it is a weak base (pKa 6.5) the unbound drug is largely (nearly 90%) unionised, so it is allowed rapid access to the brain as it is the unionised molecules that cross the blood-brain barrier. Thus when equipotent doses are given the initial plasma concentration of alfentanil is at least 100-times higher than that of fentanyl and there is very little time lag for an effect to be seen in the brain (using spectral edge analysis) whereas with fentanyl a three minute time lag is seen before peak effect occurs. Thus the half-time for plasma/brain equilibration is 1.1 minutes for alfentanil and 6.4 minutes for fentanyl.

18. WHAT DO THE LUNGS DO TO SUFENTANIL?

> ⊃ The lungs are capable of uptake, storage, release and metabolism of many substances. This topic appears in the physiology viva as 'non-respiratory functions of the lung'.

Sufentanil is a basic, lipophilic analgesic agent that undergoes significant first-pass retention in the lungs. The significance of this is that the binding sites may be saturable, and that in the presence of another, similar, compound there may be displacement of sufentanil from the binding sites with increased quantities of the drug released into the circulation. There are at least two binding sites, however, and saturation does not occur with sufentanil in clinically-used concentrations.

---

19. WHY HAS FENTANYL A SHORTER DURATION OF ACTION THAN MORPHINE?

> ⊃ The shorter duration of action of fentanyl is related entirely to redistribution; clearance is actually slower than that of morphine. 10% is excreted unchanged.

However because it is a weak base, it is initially eliminated from plasma to stomach. Subsequent reabsorption from the small intestine causes a secondary rise in plasma levels, and may be responsible for respiratory depression in recovery.

---

20. WHAT IS AN ALLERGIC REACTION?

> ⊃ There are four types pertaining to anaesthesia:

INTOLERANCE: Qualitatively normal, quantitatively abnormal reaction to drug; for example, an exaggerated response to an ACE inhibitor.

IDIOSYNCRACY: Qualitatively abnormal, but not immunologically-mediated, response to drug, e.g. gum hyperplasia with anticonvulsants.

ANAPHYLAXIS: IgE-mast cell histamine release reaction, type I hyper-sensitivity.

ANAPHYLACTOID: Direct histamine release from mast cells and macrophages, may be complement-activated; e.g. X-ray contrast medium.

The manifestations are cutaneous (flushing and urticaria), cardiovascular (hypotension and cardiac arrest) and pulmonary (bronchospasm). Up to 300 patients die in the UK every year from allergic reactions directly associated with anaesthesia.

---

21. WHAT USES MIGHT XENON HAVE IN ANAESTHESIA?

> ⊃ Xenon fulfils many of the requirements for an ideal anaesthetic agent.

Xenon is an inert gas manufactured by the fractional distillation of air. It has a minimum alveolar concentration (MAC) of 71%. It has no cardiovascular effects and it has a very low blood/gas partition coefficient of 0.14 resulting in an extremely rapid onset and offset of action. It is not flammable and does not support combustion. It is not metabolised and is eliminated by diffusion. It was first used as an anaesthetic agent in 1951 but its use has been impeded because of its enormous cost. Current work is directed towards reducing the cost of manufacture (it may be retrieved from redundant industrial equipment) and the use of very low flow anaesthetic systems. It has some promise for the future as it is not a greenhouse gas like nitrous oxide and there is a certain elegance in using something that is derived from the atmosphere and allowing it to return there.

---

22. WHAT ADDITIVES ARE ADDED TO LOCAL ANAESTHETICS TO AID BLOCKADE?

Peripheral nerve block:

Vasoconstrictors	epinephrine, felypressin
PH modifying	bicarbonate
Opioids	tramadol, fentanyl
Enzymes	hyaluronic acid
Others	neostigmine, clonidine, ketamine

Neuroaxial blockade:

Vasoconstrictors	epinephrine, phenylephrine
PH modifying	bicarbonate
Opioids	fentanyl, diamorphine, morphine
α_2-agents	clonidine, dexmetedomodine
Cholinergic drugs	neostigmine
NMDA antagonist	ketamine
Others	somatostatin, calcitonin, adenosine

Vasoconstrictors:

Vasoconstriction of vessels decreases systemic uptake. Only of real benefit when drug has intrinsic vasodilator properties example lidocaine . Bupivacaine and ropivacaine are vasoconstrictors at low doses. There is a direct antinociceptive effect by acting on α_1 and α_2 receptors, modulating dorsal horn action.

Bicarbonate:

Alkalinisation of local anaesthetics increases the unionised component, allowing faster penetration of nerves.

Clonidine:

Two mechanisms. Firstly, it has an α_2 agonist action, thus activating a negative feedback mechanism. This results in decrease cathecholamines release and modulates dorsal horn input. Secondly it has cholinergic effects, increasing the amount of acetylcholine centrally and this has been shown to have an analgesic effect.

Opioids:

Opioid receptors are found centrally and peripherally. Nerve membranes become hyperpolarised. Substance P and glutamate also inhibited. There is a synergistic effect with local anaesthetic agents.

2

QUESTIONS ON PHARMACOKINETICS AND PHARMACODYNAMICS

1. WHAT IS MEANT BY HALF-LIFE?

> ⊃ **This is the time taken for the circulating concentration of a drug to fall by 50% from one compartment.**

$$X_t = X_o/2$$

Since $\quad X_t = X_o e^{-kt}$

Where $\quad X_t =$ amount remaining at time t

$\qquad\quad X_o =$ amount remaining at time o

$\qquad\quad k =$ first order rate constant, units of reciprocal time

Substituting:

$$\frac{X_o}{2} = X_o e^{-kt\frac{1}{2}}$$

Divide by X_o:

$$\frac{1}{2} = e^{-kt\frac{1}{2}}$$

Take logarithms:

$$\ln 2 = kt\frac{1}{2}$$

Rearrange:

$$t_{1/2} = \frac{\ln 2}{k} = \frac{0.693}{k}$$

Half-life is inversely related to the rate of elimination, so that a rapid rate of elimination indicates a short half-life.

The concentration-time graph, which is an exponential curve, becomes linear if the concentration is expressed as a log.

2.   CAN YOU DEFINE BIOAVAILABILITY?

> ⊃ **Bioavailability refers to the proportion of a drug administered which is then available in the circulation.**

If given by intravenous bolus, there is 100% bioavailability. Oral preparations may undergo first-pass metabolism. Ingestion of the drug and absorption into the portal circulation presents the drug to the liver where it may be extensively metabolised, such that a diminished amount appears in the systemic circulation. This reduces bioavailability, and the extent to which this happens may differ between preparations of the same drug. Digoxin has been identified as being susceptible to this effect and the variations in bioavailability between different preparations of the drug are a justification for continuing to prescribe one formulation in preference to any other in a patient whose therapy has been stabilised.

3. WHAT IS THE DIFFERENCE BETWEEN ZERO AND FIRST ORDER KINETICS?

⊃ Zero order is where the rate is independent of the amount of drug undergoing the process; first order is where the rate is directly proportional to the amount of drug undergoing the process. See examples.

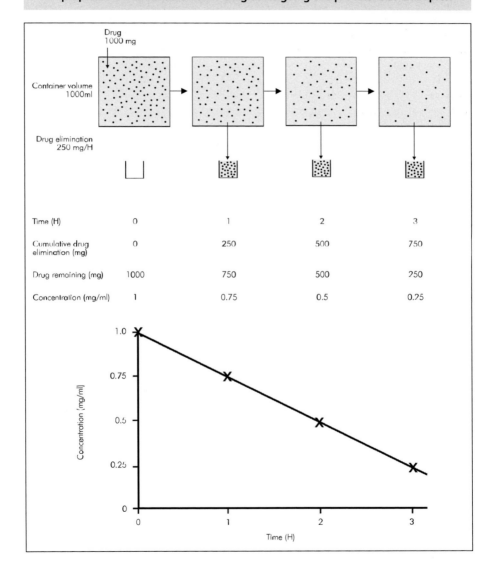

Time (H)	0	1	2	3
Cumulative drug elimination (mg)	0	250	500	750
Drug remaining (mg)	1000	750	500	250
Concentration (mg/ml)	1	0.75	0.5	0.25

ZERO ORDER KINETICS

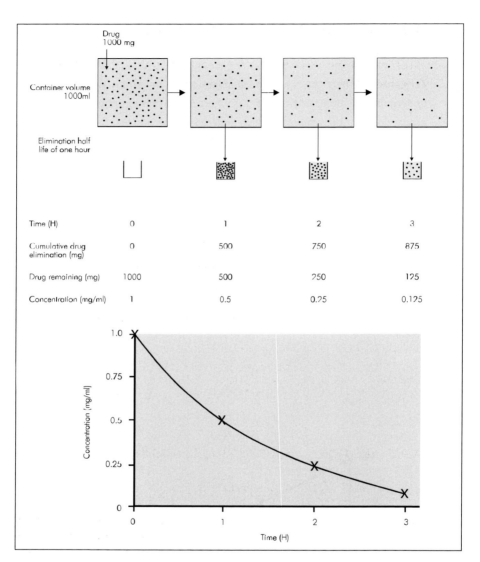

FIRST ORDER KINETICS

4. CAN YOU DEFINE VOLUME OF DISTRIBUTION?

> ⊃ This is the amount of drug administered divided by the concentration of drug observed.

Take   X   = $Vd \times C$

At time o, where Vd is the volume of distribution, and rearranging

$$Vd = \frac{X_o}{C_o}$$

In general,   highly protein-bound = small Vd

                    highly lipid-soluble = large Vd

Also,   Vd   <   3 l – drug entirely within plasma

       Vd   >   42 l – drug is distributed beyond total body water

---

5. WHAT INDICATES THE PRESENCE OF A TRUE RECEPTOR?

▪ Sensitivity: Receptor-agonist complex produces a predictable result.
▪ Specificity: Receptor reacts with one type of molecule.
▪ Saturability: The rate of process is limited by available receptor sites.
▪ Reversibility: By displacement of agonist or antagonist from the receptor site.

---

6. WHAT ARE NON-LINEAR PHARMACOKINETICS?

> ⊃ Some drugs behave differently at different concentrations.

An exmample is Phenytoin, where the clearance of the drug is dose dependent (first order) until the enzymes involved are saturated, at which point the clearance of the drug becomes constant (zero order) and so the concentration rises much faster as the dosage increases.

D_{max} =   the dose at which the curve would become perpendicular

        =   the asymptote

K_m = C_{ss} at $\dfrac{D_{max}}{2}$

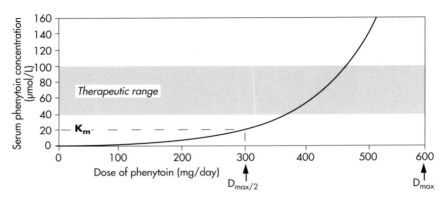

The Michaelis-Menton equation applies:

$$\frac{-dC}{dt} = \frac{D_{max} \times C_{ss}}{K_m + C_{ss}}$$

At low concentrations, i.e. low values of C_{ss}:

$$K_m >> C_{ss}$$

Therefore, $K_m + C_{ss} \approx K_m$

Substituting

$$\frac{-dC}{dt} = \frac{D_{max} \times C_{ss}}{K_m}$$

Simplifying, since D_{max} and K_m are constants for any individual

$$\frac{-dC}{dt} = \text{constant} \times C_{ss}$$

Which is a first order equation.

At high concentrations, and thus high values for C_{ss}

$$C_{ss} >> K_m$$

Therefore, $K_m + C_{ss} \approx Css$

Substituting

$$\frac{-dC}{dt} = D_{max}$$

Which is a zero-order equation.

Regarding non-linear pharmacokinetics,

1. No constant $t_{1/2}$; it increases with increased dose.
2. Area under the curve (AUC) $\propto$ dose^2 so a small increase in dose can cause a huge increase in plasma level.

7. WHAT IS A HILL PLOT?

> ⊃ A.V. Hill in 1900 drew PO_2 against % oxyhaemoglobin saturation. The Hill plot is also used to mean log dose on x axis against the response, as a proportion, where E is the observed response.

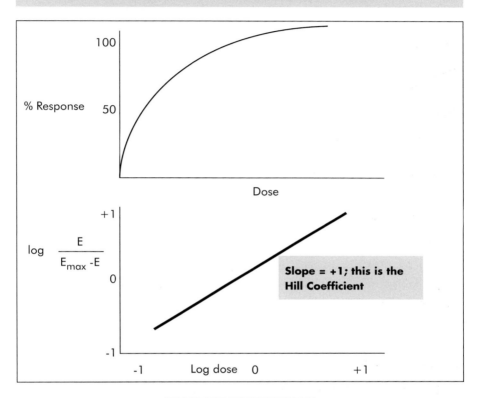

8. HOW MAY GENETIC MAKE UP INFLUENCE DRUG ACTION?

1. **Fast and slow acetylators:** The enzyme N-acetyl tranferase has two phenotypes; this affects the metabolism of, for example, hydralazine.
2. **Suxamethonium metabolism:** Suxamethonium is metabolised by plasma pseudocholinesterase.

Dibucaine number: this represents % inhibition of enzyme by dibucaine, at 10–5 M concentration. Normal is 80% inhibition. A homozygous defect creates an abnormal enzyme with reduced affinity for suxamethonium. This also happens to be resistant to dibucaine inhibition. Fluoride inhibition may also be used to further identify the particular genotype; because there are 4 alleles, there are 10 possible genotypes.

3.

GENOTYPE	INCIDENCE	RESPONSE TO SUXAMETHONIUM	DIBUCAINE NUMBER	FLUORIDE NUMBER
EuEu	96%	Normal	80	60
EaEa	1 : 2,800	Very prolonged	20	20
EuEa	1 : 25	Slightly prolonged	40–60	45
EfEf	1 : 154,000	Moderately prolonged	70	30
EsEs	1 : 100,000	Very prolonged	–	–
EuEf	1 : 200	Slightly prolonged	75	50
EuEs	1 : 90	Slightly prolonged	80	60
EaEf	1 : 20,000	Moderately prolonged	45	35
EsEa	1 : 29,000	Very prolonged	20	19
EfEs	1 : 150,000	Moderately prolonged	60	35

4. **G6PD deficiency:** This enzyme generates reduced NADPH, which in turn prevents oxidation of cell proteins. The administration of Fava beans and drugs (e.g. sulphonamides, quinine, probenecid) leads to haemolysis.

5. **Porphyria:** The key to understanding this condition is that it is due to over-production of haem precursors, which are highly toxic, in turn due to the overactivity of the small, readily-induced enzyme δ-aminolaevulinic acid (ALA) synthetase. There is a relative deficiency of an enzyme later on in the synthetic process, thus allowing accumulation of intermediate metabolites. The position of the deficient enzyme predicts the type of precursor to accumulate, and thus, the pattern of the disease, for the smaller intermediates cross the blood brain barrier and cause neuropsychiatric disturbance, while the larger ones cause cutaneous manifestations.

These are uncommon conditions, but the two important conditions are Acute Intermittent Porphyria (AIP) and Variegate Porphyria (VP). Both are inherited in an autosomal dominant form.

Both are precipitated by induction of ALA synthetase by pregnancy, dieting, and drugs of importance such as barbiturates, steroids, sulphonamides and griseofulvin. Management of an attack involves analgesia, carbohydrate loading, b-blockade, fluids and haematin solutions to suppress ALA synthetase activity.

a. Acute Intermittent Porphyria is due to a deficiency of Uroporphyrinogen-1 synthase, allowing accumulation of small metabolites: thus the picture is of abdominal pain, neuropathy, and psychosis. AIP is common in Scandinavia and diagnosis is made by finding ALA in the urine.

b. Variegate Porphyria is due to deficiency of Protoporphyrinogen oxidase, allowing accumulation of large metabolites; cutaneous manifestations of rash and necrosis occur in addition to neurological phenomena, and diagnosis is made by finding porphyrins in the stool.

6. **Malignant Hyperpyrexia:** This is an autosomal dominant condition and is associated with Ca^{2+} emergence from the sarcoplasmic reticulum. There is a ratio of 3: 1 male: female; and an association with squints and musculoskeletal abnormalities. The incidence is 1: 200,000 in the United Kingdom. The diagnosis is based on muscle biopsy, with contracture testing for 0.2 g in halothane 2% and caffeine 2 mmol/l. If positive this is diagnostic and the patient is labelled MH susceptible (MHS). The term MH equivocal (MHE) is used if one or the other produces a contracture. MH non-susceptible (MHN) is applied if neither produces a contracture, but the test is only 95% sensitive. The condition has a 10% mortality. There is an association with the ryanodine receptor gene, which is located on chromosome 19 q12 – 13.2.

IMMEDIATE ACTION DRILL:
1. Stop trigger agent and stop surgery if possible.
2. Administer 100% O_2.
3. Hyperventilate.
4. Dantrolene (modal effect 2.4 mg/kg, range 1–10 mg/kg).
5. Correct acidosis.
6. Correct arrhythmia: anticipate tachycardia and unstable ventricular rhythm.
7. Correct hyperkalaemia, and encourage diuresis; retain urine for myoglobin assay.
8. Cool; use cold fluids, through a blood-warmer containing ice; use a heating system on cold, and apply cold water to the patient.
9. Transfer to ITU and monitor progress of condition by serum CK at 6, 12 and 24 hours.

The morning after diagnosis may be made by assay of myoglobinuria, and a disproportionate rise in plasma CK. Screen proband and family.

---

9. WHAT ARE ACTIVE METABOLITES AND WHICH EXIST FOR MORPHINE AND PETHIDINE?

⊃ An active metabolite has pharmacological action at either the same or a different site as the substance from which it is derived. If the metabolite is more efficacious than the parent compound, the parent can be called a pro–drug.

Morphine: 70% is metabolised to morphine-3-glucuronide, which has little activity; however, it may be broken down in the gut to release morphine for enterohepatic circulation. Morphine-6-glucuronide, however, has considerable activity at morphine receptors and the distribution of metabolism between the two metabolites may dictate individual response to morphine.

Pethidine: Metabolised to norpethidine, pethidinic acid, and pethidine-N-oxide by phase 1 metabolism in the liver. None have significant effect at the receptor but norpethidine can cause fits and hallucinations.

---

10.   WHAT IS AN AGONIST AND AN ANTAGONIST?

An agonist combines with a receptor and achieves a pharmacological response, in other words an agonist has affinity and intrinsic activity.

An antagonist has affinity and has reduced or absent intrinsic activity.

Dose ratio = ratio between doses of agonist required for equivalent response in the presence and absence of the antagonist: a property of a competitive antagonist.

K_a = dissociation constant of receptor – antagonist complex at equilibrium, a measure of the affinity of competitive antagonists for receptors.

---

11.   WHAT IS AFFINITY?

> ⊃ **Affinity is the ability of an agonist to combine with a receptor.**

$$\text{Free Drug} + \text{Receptor} \underset{k_2}{\overset{k_1}{\Leftrightarrow}} \text{Drug} - \text{Receptor Complex}$$

k_1 = association rate constant

k_2 = dissociation rate constant

At equilibrium, $k_1 = k_2$

So, number of drug molecules (D) combining with receptors is:

$$= \quad k_1 \times [D] \times [R]$$

This must be the same as the number of drug-receptor complexes splitting up:

$$= \quad k_2 \times [DR]$$

But since $k_1 = k_2$

And $k_1 [D] [R] = k_2 [DR]$

$$\frac{k_2}{k_1} = \frac{[R]}{[DR]}$$

$$= k_d$$

Which is the dissociation constant at equilibrium, a measure of AFFINITY.

- If k_d is HIGH there is LOW affinity
- If k_d is LOW there is HIGH affinity

Similarly k_a is the dissociation constant for antagonist – receptor complex. *Liver is the*

_____

12. HOW DOES THE LIVER HANDLE DRUGS?

⊃ **Aim: To make a lipid soluble drug into a polar, water–soluble product for renal elimination.**

In two stages: **Phase I:** Non-synthetic, microsomal

Phase II: Synthetic

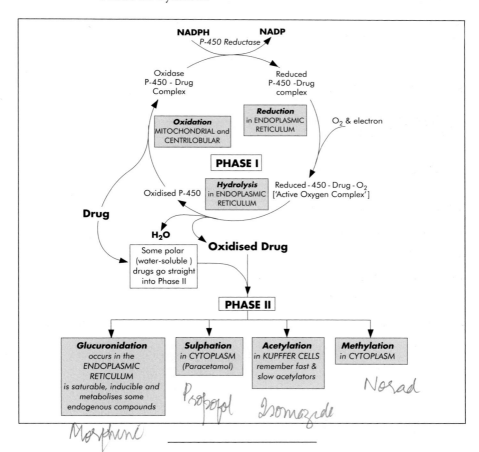

Morphine   _____

13.   WHERE ELSE MAY DRUGS BE METABOLISED?

⊃ Expect the question to lead on to a discussion of the metabolism, or of the drug, that you volunteer as an example.

LOCATION	MECHANISM	EXAMPLES
Plasma	Pseudocholinesterase	Suxamethonium, Procaine
Neuromuscular junction	Cholinesterase	
Gut wall		Lidocaine, Isoprenaline, Chlorpromazine
Kidney		Dopamine
Lung		Epinephrine
Hoffman	Spontaneous degradation	Atracurium

14.   WHAT SECOND-MESSENGERS DO YOU RECOGNISE?

⊃ As before, expect a fuller discussion to emerge from the mechanism or example you volunteer.

MECHANISM	EXAMPLE
Ion channel opening/closing	Neuromuscular junction, and the action of norepinephrine on K^+ channels in heart
Cytoplasmic receptors, increasing mRNA transcription	Thyroid hormones, steroid hormones
Activation of Phospholipase C	Angiotensin II, and the α_2 receptor
Activation of adenylate cyclase (increase or decrease in cAMP	β_1 receptor, α_2 receptor
Tyrosine kinase in cytoplasm	Insulin

15. HOW IS DIAZEPAM METABOLISED?

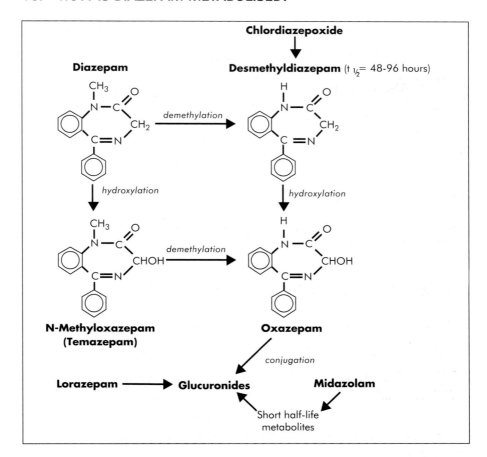

Chlordiazepoxide

Diazepam

Desmethyldiazepam (t $_{1/2}$= 48-96 hours)

demethylation

hydroxylation

hydroxylation

N-Methyloxazepam
(Temazepam)

demethylation

Oxazepam

conjugation

Lorazepam ⟶ **Glucuronides**

Midazolam

Short half-life
metabolites

QUESTIONS ON CARDIOVASCULAR PHARMACOLOGY

1. HOW IS TYROSINE METABOLISED TO EPINEPHRINE?

⊃ SODOM; Substitutions = Oxidation, Decarboxylation, Oxidation, Methylation

2. WHAT ACTIONS DO NEUROMUSCULAR BLOCKING AGENTS HAVE ON THE CARDIOVASCULAR SYSTEM?

⊃ Consider both non-depolarising and depolarising drugs.

INSTIGATION	INTERMEDIARY	OBSERVED EFFECT
Suxamethonium, which is formed from 2 acetylcholine molecules	Muscarinic (M_2) receptors	Bradycardia
Non-depolarising blockers	Histamine release	Reduction in systemic vascular resistance (SVR), a drop in blood pressure and a reflex increase in heart rate
Muscle relaxation		Diminished cardiac output
Ganglion blockade (at cholinergic receptors)	Reduction in sympathetic tone	
Muscarinic blockade		Vagolytic action; this is seen with pancuronium because of its tris-quaternary structure

3. WHAT IS A SELECTIVE PHOSPHODIESTERASE INHIBITOR?

⊃ There are at least five phosphodiesterase isoenzymes and current research is aimed at inhibiting only those that are of cardiovascular purpose.

Phosphodiesterase isoenzymes:

I   Associated with calmodulin, and smooth muscle relaxation

II   Stimulated by cGMP

III Associated with cAMP, inhibited by cGMP; causing inotropy and vascular and airway smooth muscle relaxation

IV   Associated with cAMP and airway dilation

V   cGMP specific; direct platelet aggregation inhibition (diisopyramide)

Lusitropy is the enhancement of the rate of myocardial relaxation.

Methylxanthines (for example, aminophylline) affect all isoenzymes, whereas:

Enoximone
Is a specific phosphodiesterase III inhibitor.

Presentation: Yellow liquid in propyl alcohol for mixture in saline or water.

Class: PDE III inhibitor.

Action: Accumulation of cAMP and protein kinase activity, causing inotropy, vasodilatation, renal dilation and chronotropy.

Uses: Chronic and acute cardiac failure and as a pharmacological bridge to transplantation.

Dose: 0.5 mg/kg loading, then infusion of 20 μg/kg/min.

Route: IV only.

Onset of action: Within 15 minutes.

Duration: Half-life is 4 hours.

Complications: Tachyarrhythmias.

Elimination: Hepatic and renal.

Interactions: Enoximone potentiates catecholamines.

---

4. HOW DO ANTIARRHYTHMICS WORK?

> ⟳ Although imperfect, Vaughan–Williams classification is used as a frame to demonstrate understanding. Adenosine and digoxin do not sit easily within it, however.

VAUGHAN-WILLIAMS CLASSIFICATION

I a Decreased Na^+ flux in phase 0; increased repolarisation; disopyramide

    b Decreased Na^+ flux in phase 0; decreased repolarisation; lidocaine, mexilitine

    c Decreased Na^+ flux in phase 0; flecainide

II β-blockade; propranolol, metoprolol

III Enhanced repolarisation; bretylium, amiodarone

IV Ca^{2+} entry blockade; verapamil, nifedipine

Recommendations for specific situations in adults:
- VENTRICULAR ARRHYTHMIAS:
  Lidocaine 100 mg then 2–4 mg/min, or mexilitine
- ATRIAL FIBRILLATION WITHOUT COMPROMISE:
  Digoxin 1 mg divided in 24 H, then 125–150 μg/day; or DC SHOCK (start at 50 J) after anticoagulation and stopping digoxin

- **ATRIAL FIBRILLATION WITH COMPROMISE:**
  DC Shock
- **FAST ATRIAL FIBRILLATION OF RECENT ONSET:**
  Flecainide 2 mg/kg then 1.5 mg/kg in one hour then 100–250 æg/kg/hr
- **WOLF-PARKINSON-WHITE SYNDROME:**
  Amiodarone 5 mg/kg slow bolus then 200 mg/day
- **LOCAL ANAESTHETIC TOXICITY:**
  Bretylium 7 mg/kg then 2 mg/min infusion
- **SUPRAVENTRICULAR TACHYCARDIA OF RECENT ONSET:**
  Adenosine 3 mg, doubling until effect seen
- **OTHER SUPRAVENTRICULAR TACHYCARDIA:**
  Verapamil 5–10 mg slow bolus
- **TORSADES DES POINTES:**
  Magnesium 4 g bolus then infusion 1 g/H, aim for 2–3.5 mmol/l

4

QUESTIONS ON MOLECULAR PHARMACOLOGY

1. WHAT IS MEANT BY STRUCTURE–ACTIVITY RELATIONSHIPS?

> ⊃ This is the relationship between the chemical structure of a drug and its effect. It is the basis of receptor theory described by Langley and Ehrlich.

For example, barbiturates:

- Larger number of carbon atoms increases potency
- A phenyl group is anticonvulsant
- CH_3 at position 1 creates a drug with shorter action and rapid onset
- Sulphur at position 6 makes it a thiobarbiturate, enhancing lipid solubility, speed of action and recovery.

2. DESCRIBE THE STRUCTURE OF THE ACETYLCHOLINE RECEPTOR

> ⊃ This receptor has a pentametric structure consisting of five protein subunits that span the membrane with the channel within them.

The subunits are as follows:

1. α-subunit (MW 40,000)

   ▓ This binds to acetylcholine (ACh)
   ▓ The binding of the first ACh molecule improves affinity for the second one
   ▓ The binding of second ACh leads to a configuration change, which opens the channel

2. β-subunit (MW 50,000)

3. γ-subunit (MW 60,000)

   ▓ This is replaced by the e-subunit in the adult

4. δ-subunit (MW 65,000)

---

3. HOW IS ACETYLCHOLINE FORMED?

> ⊃ Acetylcholine is formed at the presynaptic end of cholinergic axons by the transfer of an acetyl group from acetyl CoA to choline.

Acetyl CoA is formed from pyruvate + CoA + NAD^+ under aerobic conditions (i.e. from glycolysis via the Krebs cycle) or from Leucine amino acid degradation.

---

4. WHAT IS THE NATURE OF THE CELL MEMBRANE?

> ⊃ It consists of a lipid bilayer.

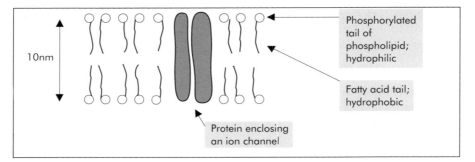

Transfer of substances may occur by means of:

1. Simple diffusion: highly lipid-soluble, non ionised compounds, e.g. alcohols.
2. Non-ionic diffusion "Facilitated diffusion".
3. Active transport: This may be primary (associated with covalent modulation) or secondary (allosteric modulation).

---

5. WHAT IS GABA? HOW DOES IT WORK?

> ⊃ Gamma–amino butyric acid is an inhibitory mediator in the brain and is responsible for presynaptic inhibition. This is to do with transmembrane potentials; a threshold potential must be reached before depolarisation can occur.

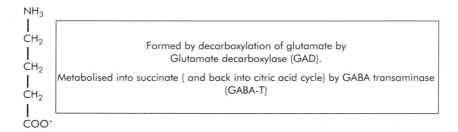

The excitatory post-synaptic potential (EPSP) is proportional to Na^+ entry, opposing the inhibitory post synaptic potential (IPSP) which is proportional to K^+ exit and Cl^- entry.

There are at least two types of GABA receptor;

- GABA$_B$ increases K^+ conductance
- GABA$_A$ increases Cl^- conductance, and is a true ion channel

The GABA receptor consists of α, β, γ and δ subunits in a pentameric form, analogous to the nicotinic receptor. GABA binds the β subunit and elicits effect. The action is potentiated by benzodiazepines.

GABA – receptor protein

BZP – receptor protein   } together form the functional unit.

Cl^- channel protein

6.   WHAT IS THE NMDA RECEPTOR?

⊃ **This is the N – Methyl – D – Aspartate receptor, a glutamate receptor in the brain whose action is potentiated by glycine, which is probably essential to its function.**

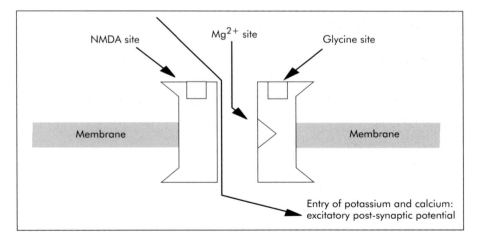

There are at least three types of glutamate receptor; NMDA, Kainate, and quisqualate. Glutamate is the main excitatory neurotransmitter in the brain.

The NMDA receptor embodies a cation channel; this causes increase in the excitatory post-synaptic potential, making the membrane more excitable and more likely to depolarise.

⊃ **Points:**

1. Glycine is required to effect a response.
2. The channel is blocked by Mg^{2+}, which only moves when depolarisation is commenced.
3. Phencyclidine and ketamine bind to the channel, like Mg^{2+}, decreasing likelihood of depolarisation. This may be the basis of action of ketamine, an NMDA receptor antagonist.
4. There is a high concentration of the receptor in the hippocampus. It is possible that it has a role in memory and learning, by means of "long-term potentiation", which is a long-term facilitation of transmission in neural pathways following a period of high-frequency stimulation.
5. It is effectively the antagonist to the GABA receptor.

---

7. WHAT ARE STEREO – OR OPTICAL ISOMERS, AND WHAT ANAESTHETIC AGENTS EXHIBIT STEREOISOMERISM ?

⊃ **Compounds that show stereoisomerism are those that have an asymmetrical atom.**

Normally in biological systems this is a carbon atom that has four different groups attached to it and so can exist in two forms that have the same molecular formula and geometric structure in two dimensions but have different three-dimensional structure. This is important in physiology because many reactions rely on the approximation of a number of parts of two molecules (e.g. transmitter and receptor), and this is based on their three-dimensional shape so this is stereoselective.

Stereoisomerism is important in anaesthesia because if an anaesthetic agent exhibits stereospecificity it implies that its mode of action involves some form of direct protein interaction, rather than a more general effect by interacting with the lipid membrane surrounding those proteins.

An important example of Stereoisomerism is ketamine. The usual form available is the racemic mixture (an equal mixture of both isomers), and its action and side effects are well known. However the effects of the two isomers are quite different. D-ketamine is four times more potent than L-ketamine. The D form is associated with less agitation and shorter recovery times. At a molecular level, the D-isomer has a higher potency on catecholamine high-affinity transport in synaptosomes, and the L-isomer is more potent against serotonin transport. Other agents that have been investigated are etomidate, barbiturates, secondary alcohols and ropivacaine.

Of the inhalational anaesthetic agents halothane isomers have been found to have similar potency, but other agents have not been studied.

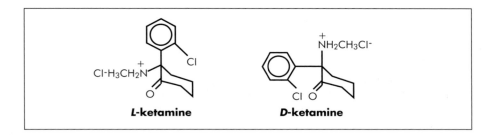

L-ketamine   D-ketamine

8. WHAT IS A RECEPTOR?

⊃ Receptors are sensing elements in the system of chemical communications that co-ordinate the function of all the different cells in the body. They are usually proteins found in the cell membrane or intracellularly.

⊃ What types of receptors do you know?

	TYPE 1	TYPE 2	TYPE 3	TYPE 4
Location	Membrane	Membrane	Membrane	Nucleus
Effector	Channel Receptor gated ion channels	Enzyme or Channel G protein coupled receptors	Enzyme (Tyrosine kinase for example)	Gene transcription via DNA
Coupling	Direct	G protein	Direct	Via DNA
Examples	Nicotinic Ach GABA$_A$	Muscarinic Ach Adrenoreceptors GABA$_B$ Opioid receptors	Insulin receptor ANF receptor	Steroid and Thyroid hormones

9. DISCUSS G PROTEINS AND G PROTEIN COUPLED RECEPTORS

G proteins:

Comprise 3 subunits α (alpha), β (beta) and γ (gamma).

The α subunit has active enzymes. Guanine nucleotides bind to α subunit.

β and γ subunits are hydrophobic and remain as a βγ complex.

G proteins are "promiscuous" and can interact with several different receptors and effectors. These targets can be:

- Adenylate cyclase, cyclic AMP
- Phospholipase C, inositol phosphate
- Ion channel regulation

At rest, the G protein exists as an $\alpha\beta\gamma$ trimer with Guanosine diphosphate (GDP) occupying a site on the α subunit. When an agonist molecule occupies a receptor, a conformational change occurs that causes the G protein **receptor** to acquire a high affinity for $\alpha\beta\gamma$ trimer. Binding of this trimer to the receptors results in bound GDP being displace and replaced with GTP (Guanosine triphosphate) At the same time, the αGTP complex dissociates from $\beta\gamma$ and it is this αGTP complex that is active and binds to the different targets mentioned above.

This process terminates when GTPase on the α subunit hydrolyses GTP to GDP. The α GDP complex now dissociates and rebinds to a $\beta\gamma$ complex.

G Protein coupled receptors:

- 7 transmembrane α helices
- Long third cytoplasmic loop is region that couples to G protein
- Ligand binding domain buried within the membrane on one or more α helical segments
- C-terminal cytoplasmic tail has sites where kinase enzymes catalyse the coupling of phosphate groups

_____

5

QUESTIONS ON THE PHARMACOLOGY OF THE NEUROMUSCULAR JUNCTION

1. DESCRIBE THE ACTION OF SUXAMETHONIUM.

> ⊃ Suxamethonium is a combination of two acetylcholine molecules joined at their acetyl groups, and this is a hint at its action. It is in fact an agonist.

It acts by mimicking the action of acetylcholine at the post-synaptic receptor at the neuromuscular junction. Unlike ACh, it is not metabolised at the neuromuscular junction but in the plasma and so the block persists until the suxamethonium diffuses out of the neuromuscular junction to be metabolised.

2. WHAT ARE THE ADVERSE EFFECTS OF SUXAMETHONIUM?

> ⊃ A very common question. Be ready to produce a list, and then discuss one of the adverse effects in detail.

- Muscle pain: This is extremely common and due to the intense fasciculations seen especially in the young and fit patient
- Bradycardia: Especially marked on the second dose – a muscarinic effect
- Hypotension: This is due to histamine release, muscle relaxation and bradycardia
- Malignant hyperpyrexia. A whole question in its own right
- Raised intraocular pressure: Sustained contracture in the extra-ocular muscles may cause extrusion of eye contents in the penetrating eye injury
- Increased gastric and intestinal secretion and movement
- Prolonged paralysis
- Dual block: This is associated with myasthenia, the Eaton-Lambert syndrome, and concurrent use of anticholinesterases including those present in eye drops
- Death: Anaphylaxis is relatively common, although death need not be a consequence
- Hyperkalaema: This is a consequence of receptor proliferation, and is seen in burns, tetanus and in upper motor neurone lesions. It is also seen in myotonia dystrophica

3. HOW DOES NEOSTIGMINE ACT TO REVERSE NEUROMUSCULAR BLOCK?

⊃ The chemical structure of neostigmine resembles that of acetylcholine (ACh), and the acetylcholinesterase enzyme has two binding sites –anionic and esteratic:

The anionic site binds the cationic part of acetylcholine, and of neostigmine.

The esteratic site binds the terminal carbon atom by forming a covalent bond, serine transferring H^+ to histidine in order for this to take place.

Neostigmine binds to acetylcholininesterase (AChE) and the phenol group is broken away, leaving both binding sites occupied by fragments: the resulting molecule has a $t_{1/2}$ of 40 minutes.

1. Thus ACh metabolism is impaired
2. ACh accumulates
3. The non-depolarising, competitive neuromuscular blocker is displaced
4. Neuromuscular transmission is restored

4. WHAT DRUGS MODIFY THE ACTION OF NON–DEPOLARISING NEUROMUSCULAR BLOCKERS?

⊃ The actions of non–depolarising blockers are reversed by anticholinesterases such as neostigmine; but the effects may be enhanced by high dose neostigmine.

- Aminoglycosides and steroids: These theoretically enhance effects, but this is rarely seen. The effect is related to presynaptic calcium transport.
- Lithium and local anaesthetics: These enhance effects of neuromuscular blockade, by causing a degree of sodium channel block.
- Volatile agents: These enhance neuromuscular blockade, by central depression of reflexes and also by direct action at the neuromuscular junction.
- Doxapram: This retards the neostigmine-induced antagonism of vecuronium.

## 5.	HOW MAY ANTIBIOTICS INTERFERE WITH NEUROMUSCULAR BLOCK?

⊃ This is largely a question about aminoglycosides, especially streptomycin and neomycin.

These antibiotics will enhance neuromuscular blockade, but they are infrequently used in current practice. Historically streptomycin was used for the chemotherapy of tuberculosis, and it prolonged the action of neuromuscular blockade. It was especially difficult to reverse neuromuscular blockade when the agent was present. There was a particular problem with streptomycin when administered intraperitoneally; the effect is thought to be due to impedance of Ca^{2+} transport. There may be a neostigmine-resistant block, which in turn can be antagonised by Ca^{2+} salts.

## 6.	WHAT HAPPENS IF YOU GIVE MIVACURIUM AFTER SUXAMETHONIUM?

⊃ The dose of any non–depolarising neuromuscular blocker needs to be reduced following the prior administration of suxamethonium. By contrast, the administration of a non–depolarising neuromuscular blocker prior to the use of suxamethonium has an antagonistic effect on the development of a depolarising block.

The interesting thing about mivacurium, however, is that it is metabolised in the plasma by pseudocholinesterase, at a rate 70% of that of suxamethonium. However, administration of mivacurium prior to suxamethonium, as with other non-depolarising agents, antagonises the development of suxamethonium depolarising block.

6

QUESTIONS ON NON-ANAESTHETIC DRUGS

1. WHAT IS THE MECHANISM OF ACTION OF ANTIBIOTICS?

> ⊃ These depend on finding a difference between human and bacterial systems; they can be bactericidal or bacteriostatic.

1. Cephalosporins and penicillins inhibit enzymes producing bacterial cell walls
2. Polymyxin and nystatin attach to sterols in fungal cell membranes
3. Sulphonamides act as false substrate by mimicking folate
4. Aminoglycosides and erythromycin inhibit protein synthesis by causing the misreading of RNA
5. Metronidazole inhibits DNA synthesis

2. CAN YOU CLASSIFY THE DIURETICS?

> ⊃ Make sure you have a sytematic frame to use.

1. Osmotic diuretics – e.g. mannitol: These agents reduce water and electrolyte reabsorption in the proximal convoluted tubule. These are used to reduce intracranial pressure and in certain cases of poisoning. In the management of raised intracranial pressure, mannitol creates an osmotic gradient across the blood-brain barrier and so reduces brain oedema. The diuretic effect follows.
2. Loop diuretics – e.g. frusemide: These inhibit Cl⁻ (and Na⁺) absorption in the thick ascending loop of Henle, and are the most commonly used diuretics.
3. Thiazide diuretics – e.g. chlorothiazide: These inhibit sodium reabsorption in the distal convoluted tubule. These are used in the treatment of hypertension.
4. Carbonic anhydrase inhibitor: Acetazolamide. This is principally used to reduce intraocular pressure rather than as a diuretic.
5. Potassium sparing: Amiloride: This works as do the thiazides, but also inhibits potassium secretion in the distal convoluted tubule as well.
6. Aldosterone antagonists: Spironolactone. The main use of this drug is in the treatment of hyperaldosteronism and other manifestations of chronic renal failure.

3.   WHAT ARE THE PROBLEMS OF THIAZIDE DIURETICS?

⊃ **These are still widely prescribed and it is helpful to be familiar with their problems.**

- Thiazides are diabetogenic
- They cause an increase in serum urea
- They are associated with an increase in urate, and the precipitation of gout
- They cause hypokalaemia, which is of considerable significance for anaesthesia
- They cause potentiation of action of digoxin and hypotensive agents
- Thiazides cause lithium retention

4.   CAN YOU CLASSIFY ANTIEMETICS?

⊃ **Best done by considering site of action.**

Chemoreceptor trigger zone:
- Antidopaminergics: these are the phenothiazines
- Butyrophenones, for example, droperidol (no longer available)
- Metoclopramide
- Antihistamines

Vomiting Centre:
- Hyoscine
- Antihistamines

Gut:
- Drugs which reduce sensitivity: metoclopramide, antacids.
- By $5HT_3$ antagonism: Ondansetron. Probably the most effective antiemetic in anaesthetic practice, but rather more expensive than other antiemetics.
- By increasing gastric emptying:
  - ☐ Metoclopramide
  - ☐ Domperidone

5. WHICH DRUGS MAY BE ADMINISTERED TRANSDERMALLY?

⊃ Transdermal administration has the advantage of avoidance of needles, but the absorption is unpredictable as it depends on local skin perfusion. The absorption will also depend on the formulation, and it may be deliberately delayed, for example with hormone replacement therapy, to provide a continuous low-dose administration.

1. Nitrates, in the treatment of angina.
2. Steroid hormones in hormone replacement therapy.
3. Hyoscine, as a prophylactic against motion sickness.
4. Fentanyl, as a premedicant for children or as patches in chronic pain states.

6. WHAT IS THE MECHANISM OF ACTION OF SALICYLATES?

⊃ There are different mechanisms at high and low dosage; this is all about prostaglandin synthesis.

Eicosanoids are products of arachidonic acid metabolism (Eicosa means 20 carbons)

Prostaglandins ⎫
Prostacyclins   ⎪ are locally metabolised, and
Thromboxanes ⎪ rapidly destroyed, therefore these are not hormones.
Leukotrienes   ⎭

These are unsaturated fatty acids with a ring at one end. Prostaglandins A and E are different families; subscript numbers indicate the number of double bonds.

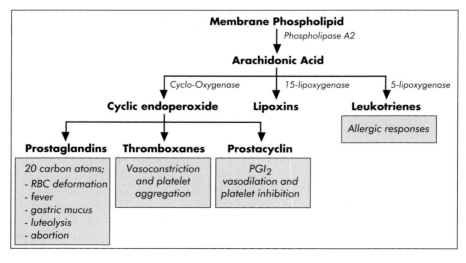

Steroids inhibit arachidonic acid release and so prevent production of all classes of eicosanoids. By contrast, aspirin irreversibly inactivates cyclo-oxygenase by acetylating it. Thus the effects of aspirin last 5–7 days, until more cyclo-oxygenase is synthesised in sufficient quantity. Therefore eicosanoid production is diverted into leukotriene synthesis causing allergic responses in susceptible individuals.

However aspirin at low dose inhibits platelet cyclo-oxygenase while sparing vessel wall cyclo-oxygenase.

So, thromboxane production is reduced, preventing vasoconstriction and platelet aggregation, while prostacyclin production is spared, allowing vasodilatation and platelet inhibition.

So: finally – actions of aspirin.

1. Cyclo-oxygenase inhibition
   - Reduced prostaglandin production and reduced pain: Prostaglandins normally sensitise peripheral receptors to bradykinin.
   - Reduced prostaglandin production and fever: This effect takes place in the hypothalamus.
2. Oxidative phosphorylation uncoupling: This leads to increased oxygen and glucose requirements.
3. Reduced thromboxane production therefore inhibition of platelet adhesion.
4. Urate retention due to diminished tubular secretion (at low dose).
   Urate excretion due to reduced tubular reabsorption (at high dose).
5. Because of increased glucose usage, blood glucose falls.
6. Hyperpyrexia in high dose because of increased cellular usage of oxygen.

---

7. WHERE DO ANTITHYROTOXIC DRUGS ACT?

1. Carbimazole and thiouracils inhibit iodine incorporation into tyrosine to form thyroxine.
2. Thiouracils and β blockers inhibit the conversion of T_4 to T_3.
3. Iodine inhibits T_4 release from thyroid cells.
4. Radioactive iodine destroys thyroid cells.
5. Potassium perchlorate opposes thyroid stimulating hormone (TSH) in the uptake of iodine by thyroid cells.

---

8. HOW DO ANTI-EPILEPTIC DRUGS WORK

⊃ **This appears frequently and is usually answered poorly. Be warned.**

Epileptic events are the result of repetitive neuronal discharges in the central nervous system involving many neurones. Anticonvulsant drugs act by breaking these propagating and recycling currents either by increasing inhibitory neurotransmitter levels or by facilitating their action by modulating the gamma-amino butyric acid (GABA) receptor function. There is the potential for new drugs to be developed which would inhibit excitatory neurotransmitters and their receptors (the N-methyl-D-aspartate agonist-receptor interaction is a likely target). The mode of action of anticonvulsants is listed below:

Modes of action of anticonvulsants

GABA facilitation	benzodiazepines
	barbiturates
GABA agonism	progabide
GABA transaminase inactivation	valproate
	vigabactrin
Fast sodium channel blockade	phenytoin

This question may be linked to discussion of the most suitable drug for the different types of epilepsy.

TYPES OF EPILEPSY AND DRUG CHOICE

Status epilepticus

First line	IV diazepam
Subsequently	Phenytoin or Phenobarbitone or Chlormethiazole or Paraldehyde

Prevention

Absences (petit mal)	Ethosuximide or Valproate
Tonic-clonic	Carbamazepine or Phenytoin or Valproate or Phenobarbitone
Myoclonic	Valproate or Clonazepam or Ethosuximide
Atypical (Usually childhood especially if any cerebral damage)	Clonazepam or Ethosuximide or Lamotrigine or Phenobarbitone or Phenytoin or Valproate

Appendix 1

PHYSIOLOGY

SHUNT DIAGRAM

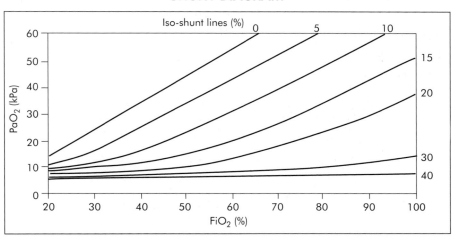

OXYGEN/CARBON DIOXIDE GAS CURVE

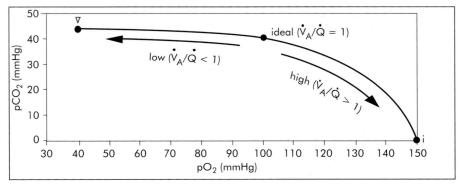

Ideal gas equation: $PV = RT$

Where P is pressure, V volume T temperature, and R a constant. At the same temperature, P and V are inversely related; increasing pressure will reduce volume.

Dead space: $V_{D\,Phys} = V_{D\,Anat} + V_{D\,Alv}$

Total dead space ($V_{D\,Phys}$) is made up of alveolar dead space (non-ventilated alveoli) and anatomical dead space (conducting airways). Alveolar dead space increases in disease while anatomical dead space increases with age.

Bohr equation: $V_{D\,Phys} = V_T \times \dfrac{P_ACO_2 - P_ECO_2}{P_ACO_2}$

The Bohr equation assumes no CO_2 in inspired gas. The normal physiological (total) dead space, as a proportion of tidal volume, (V_D/V_T) = 0.3

To measure $V_{D\,Anat}$ use Fowler's method; corresponds to vertical line through phase II of the single breath nitrogen washout. Normal = 150 ml.

Alveolar ventilation equation: $V_A = \dfrac{VCO_2}{P_ACO_2} \times K$

Where K = 0.863, if V_A is body temperature, ambient pressure, and saturated with water vapour (BTPS), and VCO_2 is standard (0°C) temperature and pressure (760 mmHg) and dry (STPD). Essentially, alveolar ventilation is proportional to CO_2 production and inversely proportional to alveolar CO_2.

This is not the same as what follows (although it is a common mistake to confuse the two):

Alveolar gas equation: $P_AO_2 = P_IO_2 - \dfrac{P_ACO_2}{R}$

The alveolar partial pressure of oxygen is dependant on the inspired fraction and on the amount of CO_2 which is, effectively, displacing the oxygen. This explains the advantage of pre-oxygenation, and explains why desaturation occurs rapidly after apnoea as the CO_2 accumulates in the alveoli unless preoxygenation has been used. It also relates to altitude, and explains the mild hyperventilation seen at altitude – reduction in CO_2 allows more space for oxygen. The equation as written above assumes no CO_2 in inspired gas.

Venous admixture: this is venous blood entering the systemic arterial circulation. Venous admixture is due to frank shunt + the effects of low $\dot{V}/\dot{Q}$. Note that while $\dot{V}/\dot{Q}$ affects O_2 and CO_2, shunt only really affects oxygenation.

Shunt equation: $\dfrac{\dot{Q}s}{\dot{Q}t} = \dfrac{Cc'O2 - CaO_2}{Cc'O_2 - CvO_2}$

Normal = 5 ml/100 ml.

Diffusing capacity:
The amount of gas transferred across a membrane is proportional to:

- Area
- Difference in partial pressures
- Constant
- 1/thickness

Diffusing capacity may be measured by the single breath carbon monoxide (CO) technique, where the disappearance of a single breath of CO is measured over a 10 second breath hold. Helium dilution is used to measure total lung volume at the same time.

$$D_L = \frac{\dot{V}CO}{P_ACO} \qquad \text{(Normal 25 ml/min/mmHg)}$$

Oxygen flux = cardiac output × oxygen content.

Oxygen content = $(1.31 \times Hb \times Sat/100) + 0.02\ PO_2$

Henderson-Hasselbalch equation:

$$pH = pKa + Log_e \frac{[\ HCO_3^-\ ]}{[\ 0.03\ PCO_2\ ]}$$

This is used to calculate blood pH, which falls (blood becomes more acid) if the bicarbonate falls or the CO_2 rises.

Laplace's law: $\quad P = \dfrac{4T}{r}$

Where P is the pressure in a bubble, T is the surface tension and r the radius. A small bubble (or alveolus) will collapse into a large one because it will have a larger pressure within it, due to the action of T in the walls of the alveolus. This does not happen, of course, because of the action of surfactant, which reduces the surface tension.

Appendix 2

PHARMACOLOGY

Within this appendix, unless otherwise stated, units are as follows:

- Molecular weight (MW) – Daltons
- Volume of distribution at steady state (Vd) – l/kg
- Clearance (Cl) – ml/kg/min
- Half life ($t_{1/2}$) – minutes

Note: Bioavailability applies to oral administration.

ANAESTHETIC GASES AND VAPOURS

DESFLURANE

Chemical name: 1,2,2,2-tetrafluoroethyl difluoromethyl ether (halogenated ether).

Properties:	MW	BP	SVP	MAC	O/W	Bl/G	O/G	Br/Bl
	168	22.8	88.5	6.35	N/A	0.42	19	1.3

Presentation: pure agent without preservative or stabilisers supplied in brown bottle with self-closing valve, which fits special vaporiser

Storage: at room temperature away from heat

Soda lime: compatible, but avoid exhausted, dry granules

CNS: anaesthesia, no analgesia, not epileptogenic

CVS: dose dependent depression similar to isoflurane

RS: dose dependent depression; respiratory irritant; increased secretions

Others: muscle relaxants potentiated; stimulation of salivary secretions

Elimination: predominantly via lungs; 0.02% metabolised in liver

Contraindications: risk of triggering malignant hyperthermia

Desflurane has a boiling point close to ambient temperature with a high saturated vapour pressure. This necessitates the use of a special heated pressurised vaporiser. Superficially this looks similar to the usual plenum vaporisers, but closer examination reveals a sophisticated microprocessor controlled unit. The desflurane is heated and the vapour kept under pressure. Pure desflurane is then injected into the incoming fresh gas, which is also heated. The system is very accurate. The vaporiser can be filled without switching off. The unit is mains operated, and is locked until the operating temperature is reached.

The low blood gas solubility coefficient is close to nitrous oxide but desflurane is more potent. This produces a rapid response to changes in inhaled concentration and rapid recovery. However, it is the most irritant volatile to the respiratory tract, and increases bronchial and salivary secretions. This reduces the rate at which the inspired concentration may be increased during induction and offsets the benefit of its rapid approximation of inhaled and alveolar concentrations. Concentrations of above 6% during induction have a relatively high incidence of coughing, breath-holding and laryngospasm (especially in children under 12 years of age), and it is not recommended for inhalational induction in children.

Desflurane depresses cardiac contractility, but this is less pronounced than the other agents perhaps as a result of sympathetic stimulation. During prolonged anaesthesia this depression is less prominent. Initially, SVR does not change but above 2.2 MAC it falls. As a result the blood pressure falls and heart rate increases to compensate. Coronary vasodilatation and increased blood flow occur. There is a theoretical risk of coronary "steal". Desflurane does not sensitise the heart to catecholamines. There is a dose dependent depression of the respiratory centre with reduced tidal volume and increased rate. The response to carbon dioxide is reduced (shifted to the right). Desflurane potentiates the effects of muscle relaxants, benzodiazepines and opioids. As only 0.02% is metabolised, toxicity is likely to be very low.

ENFLURANE

Chemical name: 2-chloro-1,1,2-trifluoroethyl difluoromethyl ether (halogenated ether)

Properties:	MW	BP	SVP	MAC	O/W	Bl/G	O/G	Br/Bl
	184.5	56.5	22.9	1.68	120	1.9	98	96

Colour code: orange

Presentation: colourless liquid in brown glass bottle with keyed filling system collar

Storage: at room temperature away from heat

Soda lime: compatible, but avoid exhausted dry granules

CNS: anaesthesia, minimal analgesia; epileptogenic and excitatory muscular effects

CVS: negative inotrope; vasodilatation with mild reflex tachycardia; coronary vasodilation; increased rate of phase 4 depolarisation; slight myocardial sensitisation to catecholamines

RS: dose dependent respiratory depression; predominantly tidal volume; increased or decreased rate; bronchodilator, non-irritant, no increase in secretions

Others: muscle relaxants potentiated; blood pressure dependent decreased splanchnic circulation; decreased renal blood flow and glomerular filtration rate; decreased uterine tone in pregnancy

Elimination: predominantly via lungs; 2.4% metabolised

Contraindications: epilepsy, risk of triggering malignant hyperthermia

Enflurane is administered using a standard specific plenum vaporiser. It produces anaesthesia without specific analgesia. In concentrations above 3% enflurane causes epileptiform spikes especially if there is hypocarbia. There is a risk of inducing an epileptic fit in susceptible patients, and enflurane is best avoided in patients with epilepsy. This risk persists for several days after administration.

There is potentiation of neuromuscular blockade, but excitatory muscle twitching may also occur from the centrally mediated activity.

Metabolism of enflurane produces inorganic fluoride ions. These peak within 8 hours of administration and are unlikely to reach renal damaging levels. However, enflurane is best avoided in chronic renal failure.

HALOTHANE

Chemical name: 1-bromo-1-chloro-2,2,2-trifluoroethane (halogenated alkane)

Properties:	MW	BP	SVP	MAC	O/W	Bl/G	O/G	Br/Bl
	197	50.2	32.5	0.75	220	2.3	224	19

Colour code: red

Presentation: clear, colourless liquid in brown glass bottle with keyed filling system collar; 0.1% thymol to protect against decomposition by light

Storage: at room temperature away from heat

Soda lime: compatible

CNS: anaesthesia, no analgesia; not epileptogenic

CVS: dose dependent depression of contractility and heart rate; sensitisation to catecholamines.

RS: dose dependent depression (but may increase rate), reduced tidal and minute volumes; bronchodilatation; non-irritant

Others: postoperative shivering is common; muscle relaxants potentiated

Elimination: 60–80% unchanged via lungs, 20% metabolised in liver (metabolites are excreted in urine for several weeks)

Contraindications: risk of triggering malignant hyperthermia; contraindicated if previous pyrexia or jaundice following prior administration.

The thymol preservative does not readily evaporate and therefore builds up in vaporiser, which requires drainage and cleaning at regular intervals. Halothane may corrode aluminium, tin, lead, magnesium, brass and solder alloys in the presence of water. Halothane is usually administered via a specifically calibrated plenum vaporiser but drawover vaporisers may also be used (e.g. Goldman).

Halothane produces anaesthesia without specific analgesia and has a low propensity for causing nausea and vomiting. CBF and ICP are increased and it should be used with caution if ICP is raised.

Halothane reduces myocardial contractility, and decreases heart rate by vagal stimulation. Phase 4 depolarisation and cardiac conduction velocity are slowed. The combination of this and increased irritability may allow ventricular premature beats, bigemini and other rhythm disturbances to occur. There is no increase in circulating catecholamines but administered epinephrine increases the risk of cardiac arrhythmias especially in the presence of hypoxia and hypercarbia. The administration of epinephrine of greater than 1: 100 000 concentration, more than 100 μg in 10 minutes, and more than 300 μg per hour should be avoided.

SVR is not affected. Blood pressure is reduced and left ventricular end diastolic pressure is increased leading to decreased coronary perfusion. This is offset by a reduction in cardiac oxygen utilisation.

Tidal volume is reduced and respiratory rate increased. The ventilatory response curve to carbon dioxide shifts to the right. Minute volume may fall or stay the same. Halothane is non-irritant to the respiratory tract and causes bronchodilatation; anatomical deadspace is therefore increased. It reduces salivary and bronchial secretions and is still the agent of choice for inhalational induction where airways obstruction is a significant problem e.g. epiglottitis.

Halothane reduces gastro-intestinal motility and reduces uterine tone. Skeletal muscle tone is reduced and neuromuscular blockade is potentiated, but there may be postoperative shivering.

Increased depth of anaesthesia reduces renal blood flow, glomerular filtration rate and urine output.

The secretion of antidiuretic hormone, thyroxine, growth hormone and corticosteroids is increased. Insulin secretion is not affected but insulin sensitivity is increased, however glucose levels do not change.

Halothane reduces metabolic rate, oxygen consumption and carbon dioxide production. 20% of halothane is metabolised and it takes 3 weeks to completely clear from the body. The main metabolites are trifluoroacetic acid, chloride, and bromide, which appear in the urine. 50% of patients receiving halothane show a temporary rise in glutathione-S-transferase.

ISOFLURANE

Chemical name: 1-chloro-2,2,2-trifluoroethyl difluoromethyl ether (halogenated ether)

Properties:	MW	BP	SVP	MAC	O/W	BI/G	O/G	Br/BI
	184.5	48.5	31.9	1.15	174	1.43	91	1.6

Colour code: purple

Presentation: colourless liquid in brown glass bottle, with keyed filling system collar, without additive or preservative

Storage: at room temperature away from heat

Soda lime: compatible, but avoid exhausted dry granules

CNS: anaesthesia, no analgesia, not epileptogenic

CVS: decreased blood pressure and systemic vascular resistance; heart rate rises

RS: decreased volume, increased rate, decreased minute volume; moderate respiratory irritant; increases bronchial secretions

Others: muscle relaxants potentiated; stimulation of salivary secretions

Elimination: primarily via lungs; 0.2% metabolised in liver

Contraindications: risk of triggering malignant hyperthermia

Isoflurane is a potent volatile anaesthetic agent, with an average speed of equilibration between inspired and tissue levels. The physical properties of boiling point and saturated vapour pressure are very similar to halothane, so the vaporiser design is also closely related.

Isoflurane causes anaesthesia without specific analgesia. It is not epileptogenic. It causes cerebral vasodilatation and there is a risk of "steal" where vasodilatation of healthy vessels diverts blood flow away from critically perfused areas supplied by non compliant vessels, which cannot dilate further. This is compounded by the reduction in blood pressure. Total cerebral blood flow is increased and intracranial pressure may rise.

Isoflurane acts directly on blood vessels reducing blood pressure by reducing SVR. There is a compensatory increase in heart rate, but cardiac output changes little. Isoflurane has little effect on contractility (excepting at multiples of MAC when contractility is adversly affected). The baroreceptor reflex is depressed. Myocardial work and oxygen consumption are reduced.

Isoflurane is pungent and causes some respiratory irritation, which necessitates slower increases in inspired concentration than with halothane, enflurane or sevoflurane, and makes inhalational induction more difficult. Isoflurane reduces tidal and minute volumes with increased respiratory rate. It reduces the responses to hypercarbia and hypoxia and carbon dioxide rises. Bronchial smooth muscle tone is reduced with increasing depth, but during the initial stages of anaesthesia the respiratory irritancy may precipitate coughing and bronchospasm.

Isoflurane facilitates neuromuscular blockade.

Only 0.2% is metabolised, and toxicity from metabolites is therefore very low.

SEVOFLURANE

Chemical name: fluoromethyl-2, 2, 2-trifluoro-1-(trifluoromethyl) ethyl ether (halogenated ether)

Properties:	MW	BP	SVP	MAC	O/W	BI/G	O/G	Br/BI
	200	58.6	21.3	2.0	N/A	0.69	53	1.7

Colour code: yellow

Presentation: no preservative; supplied in brown bottle with keyed filling system collar

Storage: at room temperature away from heat

Soda lime: compatible, but may produce Compound A (see below)

CNS: anaesthesia, no analgesia, not epileptogenic

CVS: decreased heart rate, systemic vascular resistance and blood pressure but stable cardiac output; no myocardial sensitisation to catecholamines

RS: dose dependent depression of respiratory rate and tidal volume; bronchodilatation

Others: muscle relaxants potentiated; uterine relaxation in pregnancy similar to isoflurane

Elimination: predominantly via the lungs; 5% metabolised by cytochrome P_{450}.

Contraindications: risk of triggering malignant hyperthermia

Sevoflurane has similar physicochemical characteristics to enflurane and isoflurane, but is a little less volatile. It is administered using a plenum vaporiser. It differs from the other agents in having lower blood/gas and lower oil/gas solubilities. This produces a more rapid response to changes in inhaled concentration, and speedier induction and recovery. The higher MAC (2.0) indicating lower potency is predictable from the oil/gas coefficient.

Sevoflurane produces anaesthesia without analgesia or epileptogenic spikes in a similar way to desflurane and isoflurane. ICP is raised but this effect is minimal at less than 1 MAC.

Sevoflurane reduces blood pressure primarily by reducing SVR, with little effect on cardiac output until higher doses are used. It lowers heart rate in contrast with enflurane, isoflurane, and desflurane. There is less coronary vasodilatation than isoflurane and coronary blood flow does not change. The reduced heart rate reduces myocardial oxygen consumption so the relationship between supply and demand may be improved.

Sevoflurane reduces tidal volume and respiratory rate. Hypoxic drive is reduced, as is sensitivity to carbon dioxide tension. Sevoflurane reduces bronchial smooth muscle tone and so increases anatomical deadspace. It has low respiratory irritancy.

Uterine muscle is relaxed to a similar degree to isoflurane. The potentiation of neuromuscular blockade is similar to other agents. Malignant hyperthermia has occurred with sevoflurane so it should be avoided in at risk patients.

Most sevoflurane is eliminated via the lungs. 5% is metabolised by cytochrome P_{450} producing hexafluoroisopropanol (CF_3-CHOH-CF_3) and inorganic fluoride ions. A plasma fluoride ion concentration of 50 μmol/l is quoted as the threshold for renal toxicity. Sevoflurane metabolism does produce levels above this threshold. The potentially hepatotoxic hexafluoroisopropanolol is rapidly conjugated before it can cause damage.

Compound A

Sevoflurane is absorbed and degraded by carbon dioxide absorbers. At temperatures of 65°C five breakdown products are formed (Compounds A to E). In the lower temperatures encountered clinically sevoflurane only produces Compound A (CH_2F-O-C(CF_3)=CF_2) and a lesser amount of Compound B (CHF_2-O-CH(CF_2-O-CH_3)-CF_3). The concentrations are higher with baralyme than soda lime because baralyme attains a higher temperature and the breakdown is temperature dependent. The concentrations of Compounds A and B are substantially lower than the toxicity threshold in animal studies. Possible toxicity effects are renal, hepatic and brain. A new zeolite coated soda lime may absorb these compounds.

NITROUS OXIDE

Structure: Resonant hybrid of two forms N=N=O and N≡N-O (anaesthetic gas)

Properties:	MW	BP	SVP	MAC	O/W	BI/G	O/G	Br/Bl
	44	−88	5300	105	3.2	0.47	1.4	1.0

Critical temperature: 36.5°C

Critical pressure: 72.6 bar

Presentation: Supplied in cylinders as the pure liquid (no water vapour) under pressure (44 bar); filling ratio 0.75

Colour code: cylinders french blue; rotameter knob blue; pin index 2,5

Storage: at room temperature away from extremes of heat; non explosive; not flammable but can support combustion because it decomposes to oxygen and nitrogen above 450°C

Soda lime: compatible

CNS: analgesia, sedation; not epileptogenic

CVS: increased vascular tone, rise in blood pressure

RS: decreased tidal volume, increased rate; non-irritant

Others: increased skeletal muscle activity; emetogenic

Elimination: predominantly via lungs

Contraindications: diffuses into air filled spaces causing expansion; prolonged use interferes with vitamin B_{12}

Nitrous oxide is a gas rather than a vapour (because it is usually met below its critical temperature) but merits consideration here as it is an inhaled agent used in anaesthesia. It is manufactured by heating ammonium nitrate (NH_4NO_3) to 240°C. Toxic impurities (nitric oxide and nitrogen dioxide) and water vapour are removed. The gas is pumped into cylinders and the pressure causes it to liquefy. Any volatile liquid has a specific pressure for any given temperature (the saturated vapour pressure). In use, therefore, the pressure in the nitrous oxide cylinder is maintained until all the liquid nitrous oxide has been used, the pressure then falls rapidly. The pressure does in fact fall slightly during use because conversion of the liquid to vapour uses latent heat of vaporisation, which cools the remaining liquid. The amount of cooling is determined by the specific heat capacity of the liquid nitrous oxide.

As nitrous oxide has a low anaesthetic potency, it is usually administered using a needle control valve and a rotameter marked in litres per minutes rather than a vaporiser marked in percentage. It may be administered via a Hudson mask, although scavenging is not then possible.

Rapid equilibrium of the brain concentration with the inhaled concentration occurs but the low anaesthetic potency necessitates the use of adjuncts to provide anaesthesia rather than dissociated sedation. Usually the adjunct is a volatile anaesthetic agent but intravenous anaesthetic agents are also suitable. The importance of this agent in anaesthetic practice is that it reduces the concentration of volatile agent required so that induction and recovery can be more rapidly achieved than by using the volatile agent alone. This is of limited benefit with the newer agents (desflurane and sevoflurane). However, isoflurane, and especially desflurane and sevoflurane, are relatively expensive and concurrent use of nitrous oxide makes economic sense. The reduced concentration required is also advantageous when the volatile agent is irritant to the respiratory tract.

Nitrous oxide suppresses spinal impulses and may suppress supraspinal pathways in part by activation of inhibitory mechanisms. It has a moderate analgesic effect, which may be effected through central nervous system endorphins and enkephalins. The analgesic effects are partly antagonised by naloxone.

Cerebral vasodilatation occurs with increased cerebral blood flow and raised intracranial pressure.

Myocardial contractility is reduced by a direct effect but this is neutralised by an increased sympathetic tone (α and β stimulation). Vascular tone is increased generally causing rises in central venous pressure, systemic vascular resistance and peripheral vascular resistance. Blood pressure is usually raised a little but may decrease if cardiac output is compromised.

Nitrous oxide decreases tidal volume and increases respiratory rate, the overall effect is an increased minute volume. There is little effect on carbon dioxide tension but the responses to hypercarbia and hypoxia are impaired. The gas is non-irritant to the respiratory tract but ciliary activity is reduced.

Skeletal muscle activity is increased, probably as a result of supraspinal excitation. In contrast with the volatile agents, neuromuscular function is not affected and neuro-muscular blocking agents are not facilitated. Neutrophil chemotaxis is impaired.

The oxyhaemoglobin dissociation curve (*in vitro*) is shifted to the left (affinity for oxygen increased).

Nitrous oxide interacts with vitamin B_{12} (cyanocobalamin) converting the mono-valent cobalt to the bivalent form. This prevents it functioning as the coenzyme for methionine synthase and methyl malonyl CoA mutase. Methionine synthase catalyses conversion of homocysteine to methionine, and the demethylation of methyltetrahydrate. The latter is an essential step in the synthesis of thymidine for DNA synthesis. Bone marrow DNA synthesis is impaired resulting in megaloblastic changes with metablic precursors appearing in the circulation. Eventually neutropenia and thrombocytopoenia also occur. The initial changes are seen with exposure of 6 to 24 hours duration, but in seriously ill patients as little as 2 hours will show effects. Chronic nitrous oxide abusers develop neurological damage similar to subacute combined degeneration of the cord secondary to a decrease in hepatic S-adenosyl methionine. Nitrous oxide may also have an inhibitory effect on methionine synthesis at very low concentrations (less than 1000 ppm).

Biotransformation occurs in minimal amounts. As nitrous oxide is relatively insoluble, it is excreted predominantly by the lungs. Anaerobic bacteria in the gut can also cause decomposition.

Nitrous oxide is more soluble in blood than nitrogen (34 fold). Nitrous oxide diffuses into air filled spaces (contain oxygen, nitrogen, carbon dioxide and water vapour) quicker than nitrogen diffusing out resulting in an increase in volume or an increase in pressure within a fixed volume space.

50% NITROUS OXIDE IN OXYGEN (Entonox™)

Presentation: supplied in cylinders as a gas under pressure (137 bar); liquefies at -7°C; filling ratio 0.75

Colour code: cylinders body french blue, shoulder french blue and white quarters; pin index is a specific large single pin offset from centre

Storage: at room temperature away from extremes of heat, may separate if exposed to low temperatures (0°C or lower) in which case rewarm and invert to restore the mixture;

non-explosive; not flammable but supports combustion

CNS: broadly similar to nitrous oxide

CVS: broadly similar to nitrous oxide

RS: broadly similar to nitrous oxide

Others: mainly used as an inhaled analgesic (for example in labour)

Elimination: predominantly via lungs

Contraindications: as for nitrous oxide

AGENTS OF HISTORIC INTEREST

Chloroform (trichloromethane, $CHCl_3$)

First introduced in 1847 by James Young Simpson, cardiac and hepatic toxicity led to the abandonment of chloroform in clinical practice.

CYCLOPROPANE (C_3H_6)

A medical gas that is no longer produced. Explosive but had the advantage of rapid induction, being relatively non-irritant with a low blood gas solubility, and high potency. Demand fell as a result of its expense and explosive nature. Other problems included cardiac irritability, emergence delirium, and cyclopropane shock.

ETHER (diethyl ether, $C_2H_5OC_2H_5$)

Ether still has a role worldwide as it is cheap, is stable in warm climates, and can be administered using a drawover vaporiser without the need for pressurised gases. It may be administered in air. The advantages and disadvantages of ether are shown below

ADVANTAGES AND DISADVANTAGES OF ETHER
Advantages
simple synthesis from ethanol and concentrated sulphuric acid
bronchodilatation
respiratory stimulation with increased minute volume
cardiac output well maintained by sympathetic activity in spite of myocardial depression
low arrhythmogenicity
relaxation of skeletal muscle
Disadvantages
flammable and explosive
high latent heat of vaporisation, slow induction
highly soluble in blood
respiratory irritant
slow recovery
stimulates secretion of saliva
emetic due to effect on vomiting centre and gastric irritation
may induce hyperglycaemia and ketosis

TRICHLOROETHYLENE ($CHClCCl_2$)

Used as an inhaled analgesic either alone (e.g. during labour) or as a supplement with halothane anaesthesia (e.g. using the Triservice apparatus).

Neurotoxic products with soda lime.

Trichloroethylene was distinctively coloured with 1: 200,000 waxoline blue to avoid confusion with other forms used in dry cleaning.

HYPNOTICS AND INTRAVENOUS ANAESTHETIC AGENTS

DIAZEPAM

Structure: 1,4 benzodiazepine

Presentation:

oral: 2, 5, 10 mg tablets; 2 mg in 5 ml solution

IV: 5 mg/ml clear, yellow solution of diazepam (osmolality 7775 mosm/kg) in a mixture of solvents (propylene glycol (40%), ethanol (10%), benzoic acid/sodium benzoate (5%), benzyl alcohol (1.5%) (pH 6.2–6.9)); or white opaque oil-in-water emulsion (osmolality 349 mosm/kg) using soya bean oil similar to Intralipid (pH 6.0)

May also be administered rectally and intramuscularly

Storage: room temperature

Dose: IV bolus 0.1 to 0.3 mg/kg

Pharmacokinetics:					
MW	oral bioavailability	pH	protein binding	V_d	Cl
285	86–100%	6.0–6.9	99%	1.2	0.4

CNS: anxiolysis, hypnosis, sedation, anterograde amnesia; anticonvulsant; cerebral blood flow, intracranial pressure and $CMRO_2$ reduced

CVS: blood pressure, cardiac output decreased; coronary vasodilation increases coronary blood flow; myocardial oxygen consumption decreased

RS: respiratory depression; hypoxic drive reduced more than response to carbon dioxide.

Other: clearance reduced by concomitant cimetidine treatment

Elimination: hepatic metabolism to desmethyldiazepam (active $t_{1/2}$ at least 100 hours), oxazepam and temazepam; oxidised and glucuronide derivatives excreted in urine; <1% unchanged

ETOMIDATE

Structure: imidazole

Presentation: IV: clear, colourless solution of 20 mg etomidate in 10 ml of 35% propylene glycol in water

Storage: room temperature

Dose: IV bolus 0.15 to 0.30 mg/kg (maximum 60 mg)

Pharmacokinetics:

MW	pH	protein binding	V_d	Cl
342	8.1	76%	3.5	11.7

CNS: rapid induction of anaesthesia (one arm brain circulation time); excitatory phenomena common, reduced by opioids; recovery is dose related; intra-ocular pressure, intracranial pressure, cerebral blood flow and brain oxygen consumption ($CMRO_2$) reduced; epileptiform EEG features

CVS: systemic vascular resistance, mean arterial blood pressure fall; cardiac index and heart rate decrease slightly; atrial muscle function or contraction, ventricular dp/dt_{max}, mean aortic pressure, coronary blood flow are unchanged; myocardial oxygen delivery and consumption are preserved

RS: dose dependent depression of tidal volume and rate; at a given carbon dioxide level ventilation is greater than with methohexitone; cough and hiccup common

Other: relatively high emesis rate (2 to 14%); pain on injection; venous thrombosis. There is no effect on renal or hepatic function. Steroid synthesis is inhibited, so infusions should not be used.

Elimination: ester hydrolysis in plasma and liver, inactive metabolites; 87% in urine, 3% unchanged, rest in bile

Toxicity: adrenocortical suppression when infused over a long period; suppression direct and via ACTH

Contra-indications: porphyria

FLUMAZENIL

Structure: imdazo benzodiazepine, BDZ receptor antagonist

Presentation: clear, colourless solution of 500 μg flumazenil in 5 ml

Dose: IV bolus: 100 μg increments up to 2 mg
IV infusion: 100 to 400 μg/H

Pharmacokinetics:

protein binding	V_d	Cl	$t\frac{1}{2}$
50%	0.9	15	60

Clinical: antagonises the effects of central benzodiazepines; benzodiazepine withdrawal effects may occur

Elimination: almost entirely metabolised in the liver, to the inactive carboxylate, which is excreted in the urine

KETAMINE HYDROCHLORIDE

Structure: phencyclidine derivative

Presentation: white, crystalline powder, for dilution with water forming clear, colourless, aqueous solutions of 10, 50 and 100 mg/ml; 10 mg/ml isotonic with normal saline; 50 and 100 mg/ml contain 1: 10 000 benzethonium chloride as preservative

Dose: IV: 1–4.5 mg/kg; IM: 4–13 mg/kg

Pharmacokinetics:				
MW	pH	protein binding	V_d	Cl
237.5	3.5–5.5	20–50%	3	17

CNS: slow onset of dissociative anaesthesia, light sleep, analgesia, amnesia; the EEG shows theta activity; intracranial pressure, cerebral blood flow and intra-ocular pressure are increased; analgesia is good for burns and fractures but poor for visceral pain

CVS: increases sympathetic tone leading to increases in heart rate, cardiac output, blood pressure, and central venous pressure; baroreceptor function is maintained; and there are few arrhythmias

RS: protective respiratory reflexes are usually preserved, but cannot be relied upon; bronchodilation

Other: nausea and vomiting are common; salivation is increased; uterine tone is increased; levels of epinephrine and norepinephrine are increased

Elimination: N-demethylation and hydroxylation to produce metabolites with reduced activity; metabolites then conjugated and excreted in the urine

Toxicity: rashes 15%; emergence delirium, hallucinations; pain on injection particularly with intramuscular injection

MIDAZOLAM HYDROCHLORIDE

Structure: imidazo benzodiazepine

Presentation: 10 mg midazolam in 2 ml and in 5 ml; colourless, aqueous solution of midazolam hydrochloride. Stable in water by virtue of opening of diazepine ring

Dose: IV: 0.03 to 3 mg/kg depending on effect (sedation/anaesthesia) required; elderly are particularly sensitive. IM: 0.07–0.1 mg/kg for premedication

Pharmacokinetics:					
MW	bioavailability	pH	protein binding	V_d	Cl
326	IM: 80–100% Oral: 44%	3	96%	1.1	7

CNS: slow onset of action; anxiolysis, sedation, hypnosis, anterograde amnesia; anticonvulsant; cerebral blood flow and $CMRO_2$ reduced

CVS: heart rate, systemic vascular resistance and blood pressure reduced

RS: tidal volume and minute volume reduced; rate increased but may cause apnoea; response to carbon dioxide impaired

Other: catecholamine levels reduced; renin, angiotensin and corticosteroid levels unaffected; skeletal muscle tone reduced; renal and hepatic blood flow reduced

Elimination: hydroxylated and conjugated with glucuronide in the liver, and is then excreted in urine

Toxicity: occasional pain on injection

PROPOFOL

Structure: alkyl phenol derivative, 2,6-di-isopropyl phenol

Presentation: white, isotonic, aqueous emulsion 10 mg/ml; 10% soya bean oil, 1.2% purified egg phosphatitide, 2.25% glycerol, sodium hydroxide, water

Dose: anaesthesia: IV bolus 2 to 2.5 mg/kg; iv infusion 4 to 12 mg/kg/h
         sedation: IV infusion 0.3 to 4 mg/kg

Pharmacokinetics:					
MW	pH	pKa	protein binding	V_d	Cl
178	11	6–8.5	98%	15	20

CNS: rapid onset (one arm brain circulation) of anaesthesia; excitatory movements common; intracranial pressure, cerebral perfusion pressure and $CMRO_2$ reduced; anticonvulsant

CVS: systemic vascular resistance, cardiac output and blood pressure reduced; variable effect on heart rate, usually a slight increase

RS: tidal volume reduced, rate increased; response to carbon dioxide reduced; greater suppression of laryngeal reflexes than thiopentone.

Others: possible antiemetic effect; pain on injection; excitatory movements; renal and hepatic function are unaffected

Elimination: liver and extrahepatic, unaffected by renal or hepatic disease; excreted in urine, 0.3% unchanged; non-cumulative when infused

Toxicity: a small risk of convulsions in epileptic patients; may cause bradycardia or asystole, possibly due to emulsion. It is not licensed for use in pregnancy

THIOPENTONE SODIUM

Structure: thiobarbiturate

Presentation: hygroscopic yellow powder of sodium thiopentone with 6% sodium carbonate; reconstituted with water to 2.5% solution. Reconstituted solution must not be used after 24 hours

Dose: IV bolus 4–6 mg/kg

Pharmacokinetics:

MW	pKa	pH	protein binding	V_d	Cl
264	7.6	10.8	75%	1.96	3.4

CNS: smooth, rapid (one arm brain circulation) induction of anaesthesia; cerebral blood flow, intracranial pressure, intra-ocular pressure, $CMRO_2$ reduced; anticonvulsant, antanalgaesia

CVS: negative inotropy; cardiac output, systemic vascular resistance and blood pressure reduced

RS: dose dependant respiratory depression; response to carbon dioxide reduced; may cause laryngeal spasm or bronchoconstriction

Other: splanchnic vasoconstriction; no effect on pregnant uterus

Renal: ADH, renal plasma flow, urine output reduced

Hepatic: no effect, used in hepatic encephalopathy

Elimination: metabolised in the liver at 15% per hour; 30% remains by 24 hours; excreted in urine, 0.5% unchanged

Toxicity: tissue damage with extravasation; arterial constriction and thrombosis with intra-arterial injection

Contra-indications: porphyria

ANALGESIC DRUGS

ALFENTANIL

Structure: anilino-piperidine opioid analogue of fentanyl

Presentation: IV: colourless, aqueous solution (500 µg/ml, 2 and 10 ml ampoules, 5 mg/ml ampoules also available)

Dose: IV: bolus 10–50 µg/kg
infusion 0.5–1 µg/kg/min

Pharmacokinetics:

Protein binding	Vd	Cl	$t_{1/2}$	pKa
92%	0.8	6	100	6.5

Peak effect within 90 seconds, duration 5 to 10 minutes.

CNS: potent OP_3 (µ) opioid receptor agonist, 10 to 20 times more potent analgesic than morphine

CVS: bradycardia, hypotension may occur. Obtunds cardiovascular responses to laryngoscopy and intubation in doses of 30 to 50 µg/kg

RS: potent respiratory depressant; chest wall rigidity may occur

Other: nausea and vomiting; no histamine release

Elimination: predominantly hepatic metabolism by N-dealkylation to noralfentanil, less than 1% excreted unchanged via kidneys

Contra-indications: concurrent administration with monoamine oxidase inhibitors

CODEINE

Structure: a morphine analogue (3-methyl morphine); a principal alkaloid of opium

Presentation: Oral: tablets 15, 30 and 60 mg; syrup 5 mg/ml; IV: colourless, aqueous solution 60 mg/ml (1 ml ampoules). Often combined with non opioid analgesics such as paracetamol as tablets (co-codamol containing 8 or 30 mg of codeine)

Dose: oral/IM 30 to 60 mg, 4 to 6 hourly

Pharmacokinetics:

Protein binding	Vd	Cl	$t_{1/2}$	bioavailability
97%	5.4	11	168	60–70%

CNS: less than 20% analgesic potency of morphine, low affinity for opioid receptors, low euphoria, rarely addictive, and low abuse potential

RS: produces some respiratory depression but not severe even in high doses, antitussive.

Other: constipation (used as anti diarrhoeal), mild nausea and vomiting

Elimination: 10% metabolised to morphine in liver by demethylation, remainder metabolised to norcodeine or conjugated to glucuronides. Excretion in urine as free and conjugated codeine, norcodeine and morphine. Less than 17% excreted unchanged

FENTANYL

Structure: synthetic anilino-piperidine opioid

Presentation: colourless, aqueous solution of citrate salt (preservative free). 50 μg/ml (2 and 10 ml ampoules)

Dose: IV: 0.5 to 3 μg/kg for spontaneous ventilation, 1 to 50 μg/kg for assisted ventilation
Peak effects in 5 minutes, duration of 30 minutes for smaller doses
epidural: 50 to 100 μg bolus, infusion 1 μg/kg/h

Pharmacokinetics:				
Protein binding	Vd	Cl	$t_{1/2}$	pka
85%	4	13	350	8.4

CNS: potent μ opioid receptor agonist, 60 to 80 times more potent analgesia than morphine; sedation

CVS: minimal effects even in higher doses, use in cardiac anaesthesia well established. Hypotension and bradycardia may occur particularly in hypovolaemic patients because of reduced sympathetic tone

RS: respiratory depression and reports of delayed respiratory depression probably as a result of enterohepatic circulation; high doses may increase chest and abdominal muscle tone so impairing ventilation

Other: nausea and vomiting, decreased gastro-intestinal motility, negligible histamine release

Elimination: predominantly metabolised in liver by dealkylation to norfentanyl, an inactive metabolite; norfentanyl and fentanyl then hydroxylated and excreted in the urine.(elimination half life increased in liver disease and elderly)

Contra-indications: concurrent administration with monoamine oxidase inhibitors

MORPHINE

Structure: a phenanthrene; a principal alkaloid of opium

Presentation: tablets 10, 20 mg; modified release tablets 5, 10, 15, 30, 60, 100, 200 mg; oral solution of 10 mg/5 ml, 30 mg/5 ml; suppositories 10, 15, 20, 30mg

IV: clear, colourless, aqueous solution of morphine sulphate 10, 15, 20, 30 mg/ml (1 and 2 ml ampoules containing preservative 0.1% sodium metabisulphate)

Dose: SC/IM: 0.1 to 0.3 mg/kg, peak effect after 30 minutes, duration 3 to 4 hours. rectal: 15 to 30 mg 4 hourly. intrathecal: 0.2 to 1 mg
IV: 0.05 to 0.1 mg/kg. epidural: 2.5 to 10 mg

Pharmacokinetics:					
Protein binding	Vd	Cl	$t_{1/2}$	pKa	bioavailability
99%	3.5	15	180	7.9	15- 50%

CNS: potent analgesic, agonist at μ, δ, and κ opioid receptors; sedation, drowsiness, euphoria, dysphoria, miosis (stimulation of Edinger-Westphal nucleus); tolerance and dependence

CVS: heart rate, systemic vascular resistance and blood pressure reduced

RS: respiratory rate and volume reduced, response to hypercarbia reduced; bronchoconstriction, antitussive, muscle rigidity

GIT: nausea and vomiting, delayed gastric emptying, constipation, contraction of gall bladder and constriction of sphincter of Oddi causing reflux into pancreatic duct and an increase in serum amylase or lipase

Other: histamine release, itching, urticaria, increased tone of ureters, bladder and sphincter leading to urinary retention, increased ADH secretion, transient decrease in adrenal steroid secretion

Elimination: extensive first pass metabolism, therefore oral dose 50% higher than intramuscular dose. Conjugated in liver to morphine-3-glucuronide (70%) and morphine-6-glucuronide (5% to 10%), an active metabolite more potent than morphine, the remainder demethylated to normorphine. Excreted predominantly in urine as conjugated metabolites; less than 10% excreted unchanged. Accumulation of morphine-6-glucuronide may occur in renal failure

REMIFENTANIL

Structure: synthetic anilino-piperidine opioid with a methyl ester linkage

Presentation: lyophilised, white powder as 1 mg, 2 mg, 5 mg vials for reconstitution, which forms a clear, colourless solution, containing 1 mg/ml of remifentanil hydrochloride. Further dilution to a concentration of 50 μg/ml recommended for general anaesthesia. Reconstituted solution is stable for 24 hours at room temperature

Dose: IV: bolus at induction 1 μg/kg over not less than 30 seconds, maintenance infusion 0.05 to 2 μg/kg/minute titrated to desired level. For spontaneous ventilation, starting dose 0.04 μg/kg/minute, with range of 0.025 to 0.1 μg/kg/minute titrated to effect

Pharmacokinetics:			
Protein binding	Vd	Cl	$t_{1/2}$
70%	0.35	50	15

CNS: potent μ opioid receptor agonist; analgesic potency comparable to fentanyl; rapid onset and recovery even after several hours' infusion

CVS: haemodynamically very stable; rarely bradycardia and hypotension

RS: respiratory rate and volume reduced, response to hypercarbia reduced; muscle rigidity, related to dose and rate of administration

Other: nausea and vomiting, no histamine release

Elimination: independent of hepatic and renal function, metabolised by de-esterification by non-specific plasma and tissue esterases to inactive metabolites that are excreted in urine. Unlike suxamethonium it is not a substrate for plasma cholinesterase and clearance is unaffected by cholinesterase deficiency or the administration of anticholinesterases. It is not recommended for intrathecal or epidural use

Contra-indications: concurrent administration with monoamine oxidase inhibitors

NALOXONE

Structure: N-allyl oxymorphone opioid antagonist

Presentation: clear, colourless, aqueous solution containing 400 μg in 1 ml or 20 μg in 2 ml of naloxone hydrochloride

Dose: IV: increments 1.5 to 3 μg/kg peak effect in 2 minutes
IV: bolus 0.4 to 2 mg for suspected overdose repeated up to 10 mg
lasts 20 minutes; may need to follow with infusion
also administered SC and IM

Pharmacokinetics:			
Protein binding	Vd	Cl	$t_{1/2}$
45%	2	25	70

Clinical effects: pure opioid receptor antagonist acting at all opioid receptors; effects are related to withdrawal of the effects of any opioids and antagonism of endogenous opioids.

Elimination: primarily by hepatic glucuronide conjugation followed by urinary excretion.

DICLOFENAC

Structure: phenylacetic acid derivative, NSAID; potent inhibitor of cyclo-oxygenase enzyme (COX_1 and COX_2)

Presentation: enteric coated tablets 25, 50 mg; sustained release tablets 75, 100 mg; dispersible tablets 46.5 mg; suppositories 12.5, 25, 50, 100 mg

IM: aqueous solution in 3 ml ampoules containing 75 mg diclofenac sodium, sodium metabisulphate, benzyl alcohol, propylene glycol and mannitol

Dose: oral: 75 to 150 mg/day in 2 to 3 divided doses, children 1 to 3 mg/kg/day;
rectal: 100 mg 18 hourly; maximum daily dose 150 mg
deep IM: 75 mg once or twice daily

Pharmacokinetics:				
Protein binding	Vd	Cl	$t_{1/2}$	bioavailability
99.5%	0.17	4.2	90	60%

CNS: analgesic and anti-inflammatory; dizziness; vertigo

RS: bronchospasm in atopic and asthmatic individuals

GIT: gastric irritation, dyspepsia, peptic ulceration; nausea and vomiting; diarrhoea; local irritation from suppositories

Other: renal impairment or failure; decreased renin activity and aldosterone concentrations by 60% to 70%; platelet aggregation inhibited; pain and local induration with intramuscular injection; rashes and skin eruptions; transaminases raised and hepatic function impaired; blood dyscrasias; increases plasma concentrations of co-administered digoxin, lithium, anticoagulants, and sulphonylureas

Elimination: significant first pass metabolism in liver by hydroxylation then conjugation with glucuronide and sulphate; followed by excretion in the urine (60%) and bile (40%); less than 1% unchanged in urine

Contra-indications: asthma, gastro-intestinal ulceration, hepatic and renal insufficiency, bleeding diathesis, haematological abnormalities, pregnancy and porphyria

IBUPROFEN

Structure: propionic acid derivative, NSAID; potent inhibitor of cyclo-oxygenase enzyme (COX_1 and COX_2)

Presentation: coated tablets 200, 400, 600 mg; slow release tablets 800 mg; capsules 300 mg; syrup 100 mg/5 ml; compound preparations with codeine (8 mg codeine/300 mg ibuprofen)

Dose: oral: 1.2 g to 1.8 g/day in 3 to 4 divided doses (maximum 2.4 g/day); children 20 mg/kg in divided doses (maximum 40 mg/kg/day); (not recommended in children under 7 kg)

Pharmacokinetics:				
Protein binding	Vd	Cl	$t_{1/2}$	bioavailability
99%	0.15	0.75	120	78%

CNS: mild analgesic and anti-inflammatory properties; malaise; dizziness; vertigo; tinnitus.

RS: bronchospasm in asthmatics

GIT: dyspepsia; gastic irritation; nausea and vomiting; diarrhoea

GUT: renal insufficiency and acute, reversible renal failure

Other: rashes and hypersensitivity reactions; a few reports of toxic amblyopia

Excretion: metabolised in liver to two inactive metabolites and excreted in urine; less than 1% excreted unchanged

Contra-indications: asthma; history of peptic ulceration; renal insufficiency; haemorrhagic tendencies

KETOROLAC

Structure: a pyrroleacetic acid, NSAID; potent inhibitor of cyclo-oxygenase enzyme (COX_1 and COX_2)

Presentation: tablets 10 mg ketorolac trometamol; IV/IM: clear, slightly yellow solution 1 ml ampoules containing 10 mg and 30 mg ketorolac trometamol

Dose: oral: 10 mg 4 to 6 hourly (6 to 8 hourly in elderly), maximum 40 mg/day for 2 days.

IV/IM: 10 to 30 mg 4 to 6 hourly, maximum daily dose 90 mg in non elderly, 60 mg in elderly, renally impaired and patients < 50 kg, for not more than 2 days

Pharmacokinetics:				
Protein binding	Vd	Cl	$t_{1/2}$	bioavailability
99%	0.15	0.35	300	85%

CNS: dizziness; tinnitus

RS: dyspnoea; asthma; pulmonary oedema

GIT: dyspepsia; gastrointestinal irritation; peptic ulceration; nausea, vomiting and diarrhoea

Other: minimal anti-inflammatory effect at its analgesic dose; renal insufficiency; acute renal failure; hyponatraemia; hyperkalaemia; interstitial nephritis; thrombocytopenia and platelet dysfunction; rashes; pruritis and hypersensitivity reactions; flushing; pain at site of injection; increased risk of renal impairment with ACE inhibitors; reduced clearance of methotrexate and lithium; increased levels of ketorolac with probenecid

Elimination: mainly metabolised to inactive metabolite acyl glucuronide, approximately 25% metabolised to p-hydroxyketorolac which has 20% of anti-inflammatory and 1% of the analgesic activity of the parent drug. Excretion is primarily renal (92%), the remainder in bile (6%) and less than 1% is unchanged

Contra-indications: history of peptic ulcer disease; asthma and atopic tendencies; haemorrhagic diatheses; renal insufficiency; hypovolaemia and dehydration; pregnancy; children under 16 years

NEUROMUSCULAR BLOCKING AGENTS

NON-DEPOLARISING DRUGS

ATRACURIUM DIBESYLATE

Structure: bisquaternary nitrogenous plant derivative

Presentation: clear, colourless, aqueous solution of pH 3.5 (10 mg /ml, 2.5, 5, 25 ml ampoules). Storage: in fridge at 2–8 °C, protect from light

Dose: intravenous bolus 0.3–0.6 mg/kg, infusion 0.3–0.6 mg/kg/H. Initial dose lasts 30 minutes, ED_{95} 0.2 mg/kg

Pharmacokinetics:			
Protein binding	Vd	Cl	t½
82%	170	5.5	20

CNS: no increase in intra-ocular pressure or intracranial pressure. Laudanosine, a metabolite and CNS: stimulant crosses the blood brain barrier and can cause convulsions if plasma concentration exceeds 20 µg/ml

CVS: the small amount of histamine release may lower systemic vascular resistance, central venous pressure and pulmonary capillary wedge pressure

RS: paralysis of respiratory muscles; small risk of bronchospasm due to histamine release.

Other: no effect on lower oesophageal sphincter pressure; placental transfer insufficient to cause an effect in the foetus

Elimination: non cumulative. Hofmann elimination is the spontaneous fragmentation of atracurium at the bond between the quaternary nitrogen and the central chain. This occurs at body temperature and pH, producing inactive products: laudanosine (t½-234 min) and a quaternary monoacrylate (t½-39 min). Atracurium is also metabolised by ester hydrolysis producing a quaternary alcohol and a quaternary acid. These two mechanisms account for 40% of the elimination of atracurium, the remainder being by a variety of other mechanisms.

Metabolites: 55% excreted in the bile within 7 hours, 35% excreted in the urine within 7 hours

Side-effects: histamine release may cause bronchospasm, hypotension, and erythema and wheals generally or along the vein of injection

Atracurium contains a mixture of isomers. One of these, cis-cis-atracurium is marketed as Cis-atracurium. The features are as for atracurium except as follows:

CIS-ATRACURIUM BESYLATE

Dose: intravenous bolus 0.15 mg/kg; infusion 3 μg/kg/min

$ED_{95} = 0.05$ mg/kg

This single isomer of atracurium avoids the histamine release but is similar to atracurium in other respects.

MIVACURIUM CHLORIDE

Structure: bisbenzylisoquinolinium diester

Presentation: clear, colourless, aqueous solution of pH 4.5 (2 mg/ml, 5 and 10 ml ampoules) containing three stereoisomers: trans-trans (57%), cis-trans (36%), cis-cis (6%)

Dose: intravenous bolus 0.07–0.25 mg/kg; children 0.1–0.2 mg/kg;
infusion 0.06 mg/kg/H. ED_{95} 0.08 mg/kg (children 0.1 mg/kg)

Pharmacokinetics:			
Isomer	Vd	Cl	t½
trans–trans	150–267	51–63	1.9–3.6
cis–trans	290–382	93–106	1.8–2.9
cis–cis	175–340	3.7–4.6	34.7–52.9

CNS: no effect

CVS: no effect

RS: respiratory muscle paralysis

Other: minimal placental transfer

Elimination: trans-trans and cis-trans isomers hydrolysed by plasma cholinesterase. The cis-cis isomer may be metabolised in part by the liver. Lasts twice as long as suxamethonium (24 min)

Toxicity: Block antagonised by neostigmine. Block prolonged by reduced or atypical plasma cholinesterase as with suxamethonium. Block also prolonged if factors interfering with plasma cholinesterase are present. Heterozygotes for atypical plasma cholinesterase show a prolongation of effect of around 10 minutes

PANCURONIUM BROMIDE

Structure: bisquaternary aminosteroid

Presentation: clear, colourless, aqueous solution (4 mg in 2 ml)

Dose: intravenous bolus: 0.05 –0.1 mg/kg; initial dose lasts 45–60 min; ED_{95} 60 µg/kg

Pharmacokinetics:			
Protein binding	Vd	Cl	$t^{1/2}$
15–87% (albumin, γ-globulin)	200	1.8	115

CNS: does not cross blood brain barrier. No increase in IOP and ICP

CVS: increase heart rate, cardiac output and blood pressure due to vagolytic action. Systemic vascular resistance unchanged

RS: respiratory muscle paralysis; some bronchodilatation

Other: increase in lower oesophageal sphincter pressure; may increase prothrombin time and partial thromboplastin time; small amount of placental transfer but no clinical effect on foetus

Elimination: 50% excreted unchanged of which 80% appears in the urine. 40% is de-acetylated in the liver to 3-hydroxy, 17-hydroxy, and 3,17-dihydroxy derivatives, which are eliminated in the bile. The 3-hydroxy compound has some neuromuscular antagonist activity

Note that pancuronium has some prejunctional activity.

ROCURONIUM BROMIDE

Structure: monoquaternary aminosteroid

Presentation: aqueous solution (10 mg/ml, 5 and 10 ml ampoules)

Storage: in fridge at 2–8°C; protect from light

Dose: intravenous bolus 0.6 mg/kg, infusion 0.3–0.6 mg/kg/H, initial dose lasts 38–150 min, ED_{95} 0.3 mg/kg. Onset time of 1.5 min using $2 \times ED_{95}$ which may be shortened to 55 sec using $4 \times ED_{95}$

Pharmacokinetics:		
Vd	Cl	$t^{1/2}$
270	4.0	131

CNS: no effect

CVS: increases heart rate, cardiac output and blood pressure slightly due to vagal blockade.

RS: respiratory muscle paralysis

Other: no histamine release

Elimination: predominantly hepatic but also some renal elimination. Hepatic or renal failure can cause prolongation of effect

VECURONIUM BROMIDE

Structure: monoquaternary aminosteroid, becomes bisquaternary at pH 7.4

Presentation: freeze-dried, buffered, lyophilised cake for reconstitution, containing vecuronium bromide, citric acid monohydrate, disodium hydrogen phosphate dihydrate and mannitol

Storage: Avoid light and temperatures in excess of 45°C. Reconstitution with water for injections produces clear, colourless solution of pH 4.0

Dose: intravenous bolus 0.05–0.1 mg/kg, infusion 0.05–0.1 mg/kg/H, ED_{95} 0.046 mg/kg. Initial dose lasts 30 min

Pharmacokinetics:		
Vd	Cl	$t\frac{1}{2}$
0.26	4.6	62

CNS: no increase in intracranial pressure

CVS: no effect

RS: respiratory muscle paralysis

Other: no increase in intra-ocular pressure; minimal placental transfer; no histamine release

Elimination: spontaneous deacetylation and hepatic metabolism. 10–25% of total dose excreted in urine the rest in the bile. Most excreted unchanged. Suitable in patients with absent renal function. Hepatic failure may prolong clinical effect whereas chronic phenytoin therapy reduces the efficacy of vecuronium. There are 3 potential metabolites 3-hydroxy, 17-hydroxy, and 3,17-dihydroxy. These have minimal neuromuscular and vagolytic activity, only the 3-hydroxy is found in any significant quantity and this has 50% of the neuromuscular blocking potency of vecuronium. Vecuronium is more stable in acidic solutions and is therefore potentiated by respiratory acidosis

DEPOLARISING AGENTS

SUXAMETHONIUM CHLORIDE (Succinyl choline)

Structure: dicholine ester of acetyl choline

Presentation: clear, colourless, aqueous solution of pH 3.0–5.0 with a shelf life of 2 years (100 mg in 2 ml)

Storage: in fridge at 4 °C; spontaneous hydrolysis occurs in warm or alkaline conditions

Dose: intravenous bolus 0.3–1.1 mg/kg; children 1- 2 mg/kg. Infusion 0.1% solution at 2–15 mg/min. It is effective within 30 seconds and lasts for several minutes

Pharmacokinetics:	
elimination	t½
5 mg/l/min	3.5

Protein binding occurs but the extent is not known because of the transient nature of the drug

CNS: small increase in intracranial pressure, which may be of relevance in the head injured patient

CVS: increased blood pressure, bradycardia

RS: paralysis of respiratory muscles

Other: increases intra-ocular pressure, intragastric pressure, and lower oesophageal sphincter pressure (barrier pressure is increased). Increases gastric secretion and salivary production.

Elimination: metabolised by plasma cholinesterase – complete recovery 10–12 minutes. 2–20% unchanged in urine. The elimination pathway is shown below

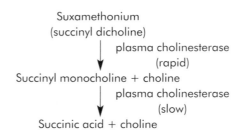

Suxamethonium
(succinyl dicholine)
↓ plasma cholinesterase (rapid)
Succinyl monocholine + choline
↓ plasma cholinesterase (slow)
Succinic acid + choline

Side effects: muscle pains especially muscular, young, male and after early ambulation, malignant hyperthermia trigger. May result in trismus, histamine release and hyperkalaemia – especially if denervation, burns, trauma or renal failure co-exist

Contraindications: malignant hyperthermia susceptibility, burns, myotonia

Suxamethonium is a short acting depolarising neuromuscular blocking agent. It is rapidly acting by virtue of rapid distribution to the neuromuscular junction and its depolarising mode of action. Its effect is terminated by diffusion away from the neuromuscular junction followed by rapid redistribution and hydrolysis. Hydrolysis occurs in two stages each removing choline. 80% of suxamethonium is metabolised prior to reaching the neuromuscular junction.

ANTICHOLINESTERASES

NEOSTIGMINE BROMIDE

Structure: quaternary amine, alkylcarbamic acid ester

Presentation: clear, very pale yellow, aqueous solution in brown ampoule (2.5 mg in 1 ml)

Storage: protect from light

Dose: intravenous bolus 0.05–0.08 mg/kg. Peak effect 7–11 min; duration 40 minutes

Pharmacokinetics:		
Vd	Cl	t½
700	8	40

Bioavailability after oral administration is less than 1%

CNS: central hypotensive effect at high dose; miosis, blurred vision

CVS: causes bradycardia and decreases cardiac output

RS: bronchconstriction and reduces anatomical deadspace

Other: increases in all the following: ureteric peristalsis, gastrointestinal peristalsis, sweating, lacrimation, gastric tone and lower oesophageal sphincter pressure

Elimination: hydrolysed by the acetyl cholinesterase, which it antagonises and by plasma cholinesterase to a quaternary alcohol. Some hepatic metabolism occurs with biliary excretion. 50–67% is excreted in the urine

Side effects: Concomitant administration of anticholinergics is essential when used for reversal of neuromuscular blockade. The increased gastro-intestinal tone may promote anastomotic breakdown. Neostigmine inhibits the hydrolysis of suxamethonium and mivacurium and other drugs metabolised by plasma cholinesterase. High levels of neostigmine at the neuromuscular junction cause a direct blockade of the acetyl choline receptor and the raised levels of acetyl choline have a depolarising blocking effect

Pharmacokinetic data for specific drugs are summarised below with the chemical structures of atracurium, vecuronium, suxamethonium and neostigmine.

PHARMACOKINETIC DATA FOR NON DEPOLARIZING NEUROMUSCULAR BLOCKING AGENTS					
	ED_{95}	Dose	V_d	Clearance	Elimination $t\frac{1}{2}$
	mg/kg	mg/kg	ml/kg	ml/kg/min	min
Atracurium	0.2	0.3–0.6	170	5.5	20
Doxacurium	0.025		220	2.7	99
Mivacurium	0.08	0.07–0.25			
	trans-trans isomer		150–267	51–63	1.9–3.6
	cis-trans isomer		290–382	93–106	1.8–2.9
	cis-cis isomer		175–340	3.7–4.6	34.7–52.9
Org9487	1.15*	1.5–2.0	293	8.5	74
Pancuronium	0.06	0.05–0.1	200	1.8	115
Pipecuronium	0.049	0.07	309	2.4	137
Rocuronium	0.3	0.6	270	4.0	131
D-Tubocurarine	0.5	0.3–0.5	450	2	120
Vecuronium	0.046	0.05–0.1	260	4.6	62

*Value quoted for ED_{90}

Atracurium

Vecuronium

Suxamethonium

Neostigmine

CH$_2$ — CH$_2$ — CH$_2$ — CH$_3$

CH$_3$ O   N

NH—C—CH

CH$_3$

Bupivacaine

O

NH—C—CH—NH—CH$_2$—CH$_2$—CH$_3$

CH$_3$ CH$_3$

Prilocaine

H

CH$_3$ O

NH—C

CH$_3$ N

CH$_2$ — CH$_2$ — CH$_3$

Ropivacaine

BUPIVACAINE HYDROCHLORIDE

Structure: amide local anaesthetic agent, pipecoloxylidide

Presentation: clear, colourless, aqueous solutions include:

plain solutions (0.25%, 0.5%, 0.75%)

solutions with 1: 200 000 (5 μg/ml) epinephrine (0.25%, 0.5%)

"heavy" 0.5% with 80 mg/ml dextrose (specific gravity 1.026) for spinal anaesthesia

Recommended maximum dose: 2 mg/kg (150 mg plus up to 50 mg 2 hourly subsequently)

Pharmacokinetics:						
MW	pKa	partition coefficient	protein binding	Vd	Cl	t½
288	8.1	27.5	95%	1	7	180

Clinical: intermediate speed of onset, long action, four times as potent as lidocaine; propensity to cardiotoxicity

Elimination: 5% excreted as pipecoloxylidine after dealkylation in the liver, 16% excreted unchanged in urine

LIDOCAINE HYDROCHLORIDE

Structure: amide local anaesthetic agent, derivative of diethylaminoacetic acid

Preparation: clear, aqueous solutions include:

plain solutions (0.5%, 1%, 2%)

solutions with 1: 200,000 (5 μg/ml) epinephrine (0.5%, 1%, 2%)

gel (2%) with and without chlorhexidine for urethral instillation

solutions for surface application to pharynx, larynx and trachea (4%) (coloured pink)

spray for anaesthesia of the oral cavity and upper respiratory tract (10%)

Dose: topical, infiltration, nerve blocks, epidural and spinal; 0.5% to 10% available; 100mg bolus then 1 to 4 mg/min for ventricular arrhythmias

Recommended maximum dose: 200 mg (3 mg/kg); with epinephrine 500 mg (7 mg/kg)

Pharmacokinetics:

MW	pKa	partition coefficient	protein binding	Vd	Cl	t½
234	7.9	2.9	64%	1	9	100

Clinical: rapid speed of onset, intermediate action; Class IB anti-arrhythmic.

Elimination: 70% by dealkylation in liver, less than 10% excreted unchanged in urine.

LEVOBUPIVACAINE HYDROCHLORIDE

Structure: as for Bupivacaine hydrochloride except: Levoratotory anantiomer of vacemic bupivacaine

Presentation: plain solutions (2.5 mg/ml, 5.0 mg/ml, 7.5 mg/ml)

Recommended maximum dose: 150 mg (2 mg/kg), total 400 mg in 24H 7.5 mg/ml contraindicated in obstetric practise.

Pharmacokinetics:

MW	pKa	partition coefficient	protein binding	Vd	Cl	t½
288	8.1	27.5	97%	1	9	80

Clinical: Levobupivacaine doses are expressed as mg of base compound whereas vacemic bupivacaine is expressed as the hydrochloride salt, Levobupivacaine therefore has 13% more activity than the same dose of vacemic bupivacaine. Animal studies indicate lower CNS and CNS toxicity than bupivacaine.

Elimination: extensive metabolism with no unchanged Levobupivacaine in urine or faeces. The major metabolite is 3-hydroxylevobupivacaine excreted in urine as sulphate and glucuronate conjugates (71% of dose in urine and 24% in faeces by 48 H).

PRILOCAINE HYDROCHLORIDE

Structure: amide local anaesthetic agent, secondary amine derived from toluidine

Preparation: clear, colourless, aqueous solutions include:

plain solutions (0.5%, 1%, 2%, 4%)

solutions with 0.03 unit/ml felypressin (3%)

Recommended maximum dose: 400 mg (= 6 mg/kg); with felypressin 600 mg (= 8.5 mg/kg)

Pharmacokinetics:						
MW	pKa	partition coefficient	protein binding	Vd	Cl	t½
220	7.9	0.9	55%	3.7	40	100

Clinical: rapid speed of onset, intermediate duration of action between lidocaine and bupivacaine, potency similar to lidocaine; may result in methaemoglobinaemia

Elimination: rapidly metabolised to O-toluidine by liver, less than 1% excreted unchanged

ROPIVACAINE HYDROCHLORIDE

Structure: amide local anaesthetic agent, pipecoloxylidide

Presentation: clear, colourless, aqueous solutions of *s*-ropivacaine enantiomer include:

plain solutions in 10 and 20 ml ampoules (2, 7.5, 10 mg/ml)

plain solution in 100 and 200 ml bags (2 mg/ml) for epidural infusion

Recommended maximum dose: 250 mg (150 mg for Caesarean section under epidural); cumulative dose of 675 mg over 24 hours according to data so far

Pharmacokinetics:						
MW	pKa	partition coefficient	protein binding	Vd	Cl	t½
274	8.1	6.1	94%	0.8	10	110

Clinical: intermediate onset, long duration of action between lidocaine and bupivacaine, potency similar to lidocaine; greater separation of sensory and motor blockade, and lower cardiotoxicity than bupivacaine may be advantages

Elimination: aromatic hydroxylation to 3- (and 4-) hydroxy-ropivacaine, and N-dealkylation. 86% (mostly conjugated) excreted in the urine, of which 1% unchanged. 3 and 4-hydroxy-bupivacaine have reduced local anaesthetic activity

Contraindications: IVRA, obstetric paracervical block; not yet recommended in children under 12 years of age

CENTRAL NERVOUS SYSTEM PHARMACOLOGY

CYCLIZINE HYDROCHLORIDE AND LACTATE

Structure: piperazine

Presentation: tablet 50 mg, IV/IM 50 mg in 1ml, and in combination with morphine

Pharmacokinetics:	
Bioavailability	t$\frac{1}{2}$
80%	10 H

Blood brain barrier: crossed

CNS: anti-emetic, with some sedation

CVS: slight tachycardia

RS: minimal effect

Others: increase in lower oesophageal sphincter pressure

Elimination: N-demethylation to norcyclizine (half life 20 hours, minimal activity), and also some to the oxide

Side-effects: anticholinergic; dry mouth, blurred vision, drowsiness

DOMPERIDONE

Structure: butyrophenone derivative

Presentation: tablets 10 mg, suppositories 30 mg

Pharmacokinetics:			
bioavailability	protein binding	t$\frac{1}{2}$	Vd
15%	92%	7.5 H	5.7

Blood brain barrier: poorly crossed

CNS: anti-emetic, acting predominantly outside the brain, but some antagonism of D_2 receptors in the chemoreceptor trigger zone

CVS: minimal effect

RS: minimal effect

Others: acts on peripheral dopaminergic (D_2) neurones. Increased lower oesophageal sphincter tone, increased gastric emptying, increased prolactin secretion

Elimination: metabolised by hydroxylation and oxidative N-dealkylation (90%); 30% in urine, 60% in faeces

Side-effects: galactorrhoea, gynaecomastia

METOCLOPRAMIDE HYDROCHLORIDE

Structure: chlorinated procainamide derivative

Presentation: tablets 10 mg, syrup 1 mg/ml; IV 10 mg in 2ml

Pharmacokinetics:			
protein binding	t½	Vd	Cl
18%	4 H	2.8	10

CNS: anti-emetic via chemoreceptor trigger zone, and by decreasing afferent activity from viscera to vomiting centre

CVS: some reports of hypotension, dysrrythmias and cardiac arrest

RS: minimal effects

Other: lower oesophageal sphincter pressure increased, gastric contractility and emptying increased, small intestine transport time accelerated; prolactin and aldosterone secretion increased; may increase ureteric peristalsis

Elimination: 80% in urine within 24 hours of which 20% unchanged, the rest conjugated or as sulphated metabolite

Side-effects: drowsiness, dizziness, extrapyramidal effects

ONDANSETRON HYDROCHLORIDE

Structure: 5-HT$_3$ receptor antagonist

Presentation: tablets 4mg; IV 4mg in 2 ml (protect from light)

CNS: anti-emetic

Pharmacokinetics:			
bioavailablity	t½	Vd	Cl
60%	3 H	1.8	6

CVS: no effect with therapeutic doses

RS: no effect on respiratory regulation

Other: no effect on platelet function, or prolactin secretion

Elimination: extensively metabolised in liver, main metabolite 8-hydroxyondansetron; metabolites conjugated; <5% unchanged via urine

Side-effects: constipation, headache, flushing

PROCHLORPERAZINE

Structure: piperazine phenothiazine

Presentation: tablets 5 or 25 mg tablets, suppositories 5 or 25 mg, IM clear colourless solution 12.5 mg in 1 ml

Pharmacokinetics:	
t½	Vd
6 H	20

CNS: anti-emetic with neuroleptic effects, acting via dopaminergic (D_2) receptors

CVS: α blockade occasionally causes postural hypotension; QT increased, ST depressed, T and U wave changes on ECG

RS: mild respiratory depressant effect

Other: lower oesophageal sphincter tone increased, anti-adrenergic activity, anti-histaminic and anticholinergic effects

Elimination: S-oxidation to a sulphoxide by the liver

Side-effects: extrapyramidal effects

ANTICONVULSANT DRUGS

Epileptic events are the result of repetitive neuronal discharges in the central nervous system involving many neurones. Anticonvulsant drugs act by breaking these propogating and recycling currents either by increasing inhibitory neurotransmitter levels or by facilitating their action by modulating the gamma-amino butyric acid (GABA) receptor function. There is the potential for new drugs to be developed which would inhibit excitatory neurotransmitters and their receptors (the N-methyl-D-aspartate agonist-receptor interaction is a likely target). The mode of action of anticonvulsants is listed below.

MODES OF ACTION OF ANTICONVULSANTS	
GABA facilitation	benzodiazepines barbiturates
GABA agonism	progabide
GABA transaminase inactivation	valproate vigabactrin
Fast sodium channel blockade	phenytoin

BENZODIAZEPINES

Examples: clobazam, clonazepam, diazepam

Benzodiazepines act by attaching to a specific area of the GABA receptor complex. The benzodiazepine has an agonist activity at this site, which facilitates the opening of the chloride channel by GABA. Chloride ions then flow down the concentration gradient into the cell making it hyperpolarised (more negative) and so less excitable.

Diazepam is primarily used for the acute treatment of convulsions. It has the disadvantage of pronounced sedation, long half-life and active metabolite. Other benzodiazepines may be used prophylactically.

BARBITURATES

Examples: phenobarbitone, primidone

All barbiturates posses anticonvulsant activity but phenobarbitone is less sedative for a given anticonvulsant activity. It binds to the GABA receptor at a site distinct from the benzodiazepine receptor area, and facilitates the chloride channel opening. It is inhibitory at some excitatory synapses.

The barbiturate primidone acts by being converted to phenobarbitone.

PHENYTOIN

Phenytoin is a hydantoin that also has local anaesthetic and anti-arrhythmic properties. It has structural similarities with the barbiturates. The site of action of phenytoin is the fast sodium channel responsible for depolarisation during an action potential. It binds to the channel when it is refractory following opening and is therefore most effective when repetitive discharges occur. It may also interfere with calcium entry and with calmodulin protein kinases. Phenytoin can cause hirsuitism, gum hyperplasia, megaloblastic anaemia and foetal malformations.

There is the potential for interaction with other drugs including other anticonvulsants. The high degree of protein binding (85% bound to albumin) results in competition for the binding site with salicylates, phenylbutazone and valproate. Phenytoin metabolism is competitively inhibited by phenobarbitone due to enzyme induction in the liver. The same hepatic microsomal enzymes are induced by phenytoin, phenobarbitone, steroids, oestrogens and coumarins. In the same manner as for ethanol the enzyme system is readily saturated so that as doses increase the metabolism changes from first order kinetics (metabolism proportional to concentration) to zero order kinetics (metabolism constant and maximal) thus "half life" subsequently increases with dose.

CARBAMAZEPINE

Carbamazepine is structurally similar to the tricyclic antidepressants and also has pharmacological similarities with phenytoin but the precise mode of action is not known. With chronic usage the half-life decreases from 30 hours to 15 hours due to enzyme induction.

Other anticonvulsants include sodium valproate, a monocarboxylic acid which increases brain levels of GABA by inhibiting GABA-transaminase, vigabactrin which inactivates GABA-transaminase by forming an irreversible (covalent) bond and ethosuximide whose mode of action is unknown.

The drug chosen for treatment of epilepsy depends greatly on the type of fits.

TYPES OF EPILEPSY AND DRUG CHOICE

Status epilepticus	
First line	IV diazepam
Subsequently	phenytoin or phenobarbitone or chlormethiazole or paraldehyde
Prevention	
Absences (petit mal)	eethosuximide or valproate
Tonic-clonic	carbamazepine or phenytoin or valproate or phenobarbitone
Myoclonic	valproate or clonazepam or ethosuximide
Atypical (Usually childhood **especially if any cerebral damage)**	clonazepam or ethosuximide or lamotrigine or phenobarbitone or phenytoin or valproate

In pregnancy, most anticonvulsant drugs carry a risk of causing neural tube defects, teratogenicity, and coagulation disorders in the newborn. Counselling, antenatal screening, folate supplements and predelivery vitamin K should be considered. The greatest risk to mother and baby, however, is that of the re-emergence of convulsions. Fears about the drugs may lead to poor compliance in the complacent patient. In addition the increase in body water during pregnancy will dilute the concentration of the anticonvulsant agent thereby reducing its clinical effect.

ANTIDEPRESSANT AGENTS

There are several different classes of antidepressant agents. The classic groups of tricyclic agents and inhibitors of monoamine oxidase have recently been joined by the serotonin re-uptake inhibitors. The major categories of antidepressant drugs are listed in below.

CLASSES OF ANTIDEPRESSANTS	
Tricyclic antidepressants	dibenzazepines bibenzcycloheptenes
Monoamine oxidase inhibitors	hydrazines propargylamines cyclopropylamines reversible MAOI (RIMA)
Selective serotonin re-uptake inhibitors (SSRI)	
Other antidepressants	Lithium

Miscellaneous agents that are unrealated either structurally or functionally may also show antidepressant activity. Amongst these are nomifensine, maprotiline, venlafaxine, nefazodone, flupenthixol, and L-tryptophan.

TRICYCLIC ANTIDEPRESSANTS

Examples: dibenzazepines (clomipramine, imipramine)
bibenzcycloheptenes (amitriptyline, nortriptyline)

Tricyclic antidepressants are chemically related to the phenothiazines, but differ in that the central ring has an additional carbon atom. This changes the shape of the molecule from the planar phenothiazine molecule to a three dimensional skeleton. Tricyclic antidepressants act by preventing re-uptake of neurotransmitter (norepinephrine primarily) into the nerve terminal of monoaminergic neurones. This action is stronger at noradrenergic and serotinergic sites than dopaminergic sites. Some drugs also act on presynaptic α_2 receptors to increase neurotransmitter release. Tricyclic agents also antagonise muscarinic cholinergic (amitriptyline is used in the treatment of nocturnal enuresis), H_1 histaminergic, and α_1 adrenergic receptors. In addition to the antidepressant effects they cause sedation, weakness and fatigue. Cardiac effects include postural hypotension, sinus tachycardia and cardiac arrhythmias. Amitriptyline prolongs the PR and QT intervals on the ECG. In the plasma tricyclic antidepressants are 90% to 95% bound to albumin, and may become displaced by drugs such as aspirin which compete for the same binding sites.

Whilst re-uptake blockade occurs soon after administration, the onset of antidepressant action takes several weeks to develop. It is not clear why this is so but it may be due to down-regulation of adrenergic and 5-HT receptors.

Tricyclic agents are metabolised by hepatic microsomal enzymes, and are therefore competitively antagonised by some neuroleptic drugs which share the same route of excretion. There are two main methods of metabolism; either N-demethylation converting the tertiary amine to a secondary amine, or ring hydroxylation.

MONOAMINE OXIDASE INHIBITORS (MAOI)

Examples: hydrazines (iproniazid, phenelzine)
propargylamines (pargyline, selegiline)
cyclopropylamines (tranylcypromine)

Two variants of monoamine oxidase have been described (MAO-A and MAO-B). MAO-A is more effective at oxidising norepinephrine and 5-HT than MAO-B but types A and B are equally effective in the metabolism of dopamine and tyramine. Antidepressant activity is conferred by inhibition of MAO-A. MAOI's act by antagonising the breakdown of monoamine neurotransmitters after uptake into the nerve terminal.

The classical MAOIs are irreversible (although a new class of reversible MAOIs now exists). Pargyline, phenelzine, tranylcypromine and iproniazid non-selectively inhibit both MAO-A and MAO-B, while clorygyline is selective for MAO-A. Selegiline is selective for MAO-B and is therefore not antidepressant, but is used in Parkinsonism acting by inhibition of dopamine oxidation. Re-uptake blockade occurs soon after administration, but the onset of antidepressant action takes several weeks to develop. In a similar fashion to the tricyclic antidepressants this may be due to down-regulation of adrenergic and 5-HT receptors. Patients being treated with MAOI drugs also become compromised in their ability to metabolise exogenously administered amines. The pressor effect of tyramine (which is found in cheese, broad beans, red wine and marmite) is greatly enhanced. Indirect sympathomimetic drugs such as those found in cough medicines will show enhanced effects. A specific interaction with pethidine may result in profound coma.

REVERSIBLE MAOIs

Example: moclobemide.

These drugs reversibly inhibit MAO-A (also called RIMA – Reversible Inhibition of MAO-A). Caution should still be exercised with foods rich in tyramine, and sympathomimetic agents but the problem is likely to be less marked. The advantage of RIMAs is that they can be stopped and another antidepressant started without the need to wait several weeks for MAO enzyme regeneration.

SELECTIVE SEROTONIN REUPTAKE INHIBITORS (SSRI)

Examples: fluoxetine, paroxetine, sertraline

SSRI's act by increasing the level of 5-HT at the neuronal receptors. The specificity for 5-HT results in fewer anti muscarinic and cardiac side effects than other antidepressants. Sedation is less marked than with the tricyclic antidepressants.

Diarrhoea, nausea and vomiting are more common, and headache, restlessness, and anxiety mayalso occur. Withdrawal should be slow, over several weeks and MAOI therapy should not be started until 2 to 5 weeks after stopping the SSRI treatment (dependent on which drug was being taken). SSRI should not be started until 2 weeks after stopping MAOI therapy.

LITHIUM

Lithium is used prophylactically to suppress the manic element of bipolar depression (manic-depressive psychosis). It is unclear how the pharmacological activity of lithium produces the clinical effect. The active component of lithium carbonate is the lithium cation (Li^+).

Chemically lithium is the first element in group IA of the periodic table (same group as sodium and potassium). It has the atomic number 3 and a molecular weight of 7. It mimics cations, especially sodium. It passes through the fast sodium channels easily being smaller, but the sodium/potassium ATPase pump does not readily extract lithium from the cells, and it therefore tends to accumulate intracellularly which in turn displaces potassium and reduces the outward leakage of potassium which is responsible for maintaining the negative intracellular potential. In this way the transmembrane potential becomes reduced and neuronal depolarisation is facilitated. Lithium also reduces brain levels of norepinephrine and 5-HT acutely, reduces cyclic AMP production, and reduces inositol triphosphate.

Lithium has a low therapeutic index and plasma levels should therefore be maintained between 0.8 and 1.2 mmol/l. Toxicity occurs with levels of 2.0 mmol/l and above. The half-life of the extracellular ion is about 12 hours and lithium should be stopped 2 to 3 days before using a muscle relaxant drug. This is particularly important for non-depolarising relaxants, which are potentiated. It may also delay the onset and prolong relaxation with suxamethonium. The intracellular lithium takes a further 1 to 2 weeks to excrete. Lithium inhibits antidiuretic hormone (ADH) activity in the kidney via cyclic AMP and increases aldosterone secretion, which can result in renal tubular damage. Thyroid hypertrophy and hypothyroidism may occur. Neurological effects include thirst, tremor, muscle weakness, confusion and seizures. Cardiac arrhythmias may be induced and all toxic effects are enhanced if dehydration occurs. Close monitoring of clinical state, lithium levels and renal function is essential to minimise toxicity.

ANTIPSYCHOTIC DRUGS

A wide variety of drugs have antipsychotic activity. These have been variously referred to as neuroleptics, major tranquillisers and antischizophrenia drugs. Specific categories of drug that have antipsychotic acivity include the following:

- phenothiazines
- butyrophenones
- thioxanthines
- benzamide

- diphenylbutylpiperazine
- dibenzodiazepines

The mode of action of these drugs in the treatment of psychosis is not precisely known. Various receptor systems have been implicated including dopaminergic, noradrenergic and 5-hydroxytryptaminergic (serotonergic). It is likely that many different receptors are affected, but D_2 dopaminergic receptors are currently thought to be the most important. Whilst D_1 receptors increase adenylate cyclase activity generally, D_2 receptors are found both pre- and post-synaptically and blocking potency at these receptors correlates closely with clinical potency. The delay in onset of a therapeutic effect from these drugs may in part be explained by a slow increase in the numbers of D_2 receptors over several weeks. Some antipsychotic drugs are formulated so that they may be administered by deep intramuscular injection given at intervals of one to four weeks.

As antipsychotic agents affect so many receptors, a wide diversity of adverse effects results. These are listed in below.

PHENOTHIAZINES

ADVERSE EFFECTS OF ANTIPSYCHOTIC DRUGS	
Anti dopaminergic	antiemesis extrapyramidal features: facial grimacing involuntary movements of tongue and limbs oculogyric crises torsion spasms tasikinesia akithisia Parkinsonism tardive dyskinesia increased prolactin secretion
Anti muscarinic	dry mouth urinary retention blurred vision precipitation of glaucoma
Anti-a adrenergic	postural hypotension
Anti histaminergic	sedation

Phenothiazines may be classified chemically by the side chain on the nitrogen atom of the phenothiazine base as follows:

- aliphatic chlorpromazine
- piperazine fluphenazine
- piperidine thioridazine

The side chains alter the potency and specificity for the receptor types and in turn alter the clinical features (see below).

RECEPTOR SENSITIVITY OF PHENOTHIAZINES					
Chain	Receptor blockade			Clinical effect	
	D_2	Alpha adrenergic	Muscarinic	Extrapyramidal	Sedation
Aliphatic	+	+++	++	++	+++
Piperidine	++	++	+++	+	++
Piperazine	+++	+	+	+++	+

THIOXANTHINES

Examples: flupenthixol, zuclopenthixol.

Thioxanthines are similar in structure and function to the aliphatic phenothiazines, and therefore block D_2 receptors more than D_1. Flupenthixol is also employed clinically as an antidepressant agent.

Other miscellaneous antipsychotic drugs include: sulpiride, which has a greater affinity for D_2 than D_1 receptors, Pimozide which may prolong QT interval on the ECG and clozapine which has been associated with agranulocytosis.

ANTI-PARKINSONIAN DRUGS

Parkinson's disease is caused by a dysfunction within the basal ganglia. The predominant change is a deficit of dopamine with an increase in dopamine D_2 receptors but other neurotransmitters are also implicated in the pathology of the disease. Drugs that affect Parkinson's disease may act in any of the following ways:

- increased dopamine synthesis (Levodopa)
- decreased peripheral conversion of L-DOPA (carbidopa)
- decreased dopamine breakdown (selegiline)
- dopamine receptor antagonists (bromocriptine)
- dopamine receptor facilitators (amantadine)
- acetyl choline antagonists (benztropine)

LEVODOPA

Levodopa is used to increase brain levels of dopamine. Dopamine itself does not cross the blood-brain barrier, and racemic DOPA produces numerous systemic side effects without being effective. DOPA is well absorbed orally and 95% is converted into dopamine by DOPA-decarboxylase. This is then metabolised by monoamine oxidase and catechol-o-methyl transferase (COMT). About 1% of the drug enters the brain where it is converted into its active form, dopamine. Levodopa causes an increase in the number of dopamine (D_2) receptors in the brain.

CARBIDOPA

Used in conjunction with levodopa, carbidopa increases the proportion of the oral dose of levodopa entering the brain by inhibiting its peripheral conversion to dopamine. Carbidopa itself does not cross the blood-brain barrier and therefore does not interfere with subsequent conversion in the brain

DOMPERIDONE

Used in conjunction with levodopa, this dopamine antagonist only crosses the blood-brain barrier slowly and is used to reduce the peripheral effects of dopamine. It has important anti-emetic activity peripherally and also at the chemoreceptor trigger zone. Domperidone permits the use of larger doses of levodopa than would otherwise be possible without gross unwanted effects.

SELEGILINE

Selegiline is a selective MAO-B inhibitor. This selectivity reduces the peripheral effects of conventional MAO inhibitors, which are largely due to MAO-A inhibition. There is no effect from tyramine containing foods and drug interactions are less severe and less common.

BROMOCRIPTINE

Bromocryptine acts by direct stimulation of central dopamine (D_2) receptors. They are reserved for patients in whom levodopa is ineffective. Predictably these drugs inhibit prolactin secretion. Bromocriptine is chemically related to the ergot alkaloids. It is often referred to as a 'dopamine facilitator'.

AMANTIDINE

The mode of action of amantidine remains obscure. Possibilities include faciltation of dopamine release, inhibition of dopamine metabolism and direct D_2 agonist activity.

ACETYL CHOLINE ANTAGONISTS

Examples: benzhexol, benztropine, orphenadrine, procyclidine

Certain muscarinic antagonists are able to cross the blood brain barrier having a preferential action on central muscarinic receptors thus minimising their peripheral side effects. The central excitatory effects of acetyl choline are inhibited and this may restore the imbalance between cholinergic and dopaminergic activity which occurs in Parkinson's disease. Cholinergic antagonists also antagonise presynaptic inhibition of dopaminergic neurones so increasing dopamine release, which may prove therapeutic.

AUTONOMIC NERVOUS SYSTEM PHARMACOLOGY

EPINEPHRINE

Structure: catecholamine; α and β agonist

Preparation: IV/SC: 1 mg in 1 ml (1 in 1000) and 1 mg in 10 ml (1 in 10 000); also added to local anaesthetics 1: 200 000 (1 mg in 200 ml)

Dose: highly variable depending upon indication and route

CNS: limited crossing of the blood brain barrier but does cause excitation. Neuromuscular transmission facilitated

CVS: heart rate increased (may be reflexly reduced); contractility, stroke volume and cardiac oxygen consumption increased; systemic vasoconstriction but vasodilatation in skeletal muscle; mean arterial pressure, systolic and pulse pressure increased, diastolic decreased; coronary blood flow increased

RS: bronchodilatation; respiratory rate and tidal volume increased; secretions more tenacious

Other: gastro-intestinal tract tone and secretions decreased, splanchnic blood flow decreased; renal blood flow increased; bladder tone reduced but sphincter tone increased; clotting factor V increased leading to enhanced platelet aggregation and coagulation; metabolic effects to increase gluconeogenesis and increase metabolic rate

Metabolism: by catechol-O-methyl transferease (COMT) in the liver and monoamine oxidase (MAO) in adrenergic neurones to inactive metabolites 3-methoxy-4-hydroxy phenylethylene and 3-methoxy-4-hydroxy mandelic acid

Contra-indications: beware arrythmias with halothane; caution with MAO inhibitors

Toxicity: there are many adverse effects but the major ones are cardiac; increases cardiac sensitivity and irritability so arrythmias including VF and asystole are likely if given too quickly

DOBUTAMINE HYDROCHLORIDE

Structure: catecholamine; β_1 and β_2 (and α_1) agonist

Preparation: 250 mg dobutamine and 4.8 mg sodium metabisulphite in 20 ml for further dilution prior to administration

Dose: infusion 0.5 – 40 μg/kg/min

CNS: stimulant at high dose

CVS: heart rate, stroke volume, cardiac output increased, atrioventricular node conduction enhanced; vasodilatation; systemic vascular resistance and left ventricular end-diastolic pressure (LVEDP) reduced; coronary perfusion may increase

RS: no effect

Other: β_1 effect increases renin output; urine output increases secondary to increased cardiac output

Metabolism: converted to 3-O-methyldobutamine by COMT; this is conjugated and excreted in urine (80%) and faeces (20%)

Contra-indications: increasing doses cause tachycardia, hypertension, and arrrythmias; angina may occur in susceptible patients; allergic reactions to the metabisulphite preservative have occurred

DOPAMINE

Structure: catecholamine; β, and α agonist

Preparation: 400 mg (1600 μg/ml) and 800 mg (3200 μg/ml) in 250 ml 5% dextrose (other mixtures available)

Dose: intravenous infusion: 1 to 20 μg/kg/min
1 to 5 μg/kg/min increases renal blood flow
5 to 15 μg/kg/min inotropic
15 to 20 μg/kg/min vasoconstricts

L-dopamine crosses the blood brain barrier but not D-dopamine. Dopamine causes nausea by its action on D_2 receptors in the chemoreceptor trigger zone

CVS: contractility, stroke volume increased; little effect on heart rate; systemic vascular resistance, systolic, mean and diastolic blood pressures decreased; coronary blood flow increased

RS: carotid bodies stimulated leading to reduced respiratory response to hypoxia

Other: splanchnic (including renal) vasodilatation; renal blood flow, glomerular filtrate, urine (volume and sodium content) increased; prolactin secretion inhibited (also known as prolactin inhibiting hormone (PIH) secreted by the posterior pituitary)

Metabolism: by COMT and MAO to homovanillic acid and 3,4-dihydroxyphenylacetic acid. Predominantly excreted in urine conjugated and unconjugated; 25% of the dopamine is taken up into adrenergic nerve endings and is converted to norepinephrine

Contra-indications: nausea, tachycardia and dysrrhythmias; caution with MAO inhibitors

DOPEXAMINE HYDROCHLORIDE

Structure: catecholamine; dopamine (D_1 and D_2) and β_2 agonist

Preparation: colourless, aqueous solution adjusted to a pH of 2.5, containing 50mg dopexamine hydrochloride in 5 ml, and 0.01% disodium edetate; requires dilution prior to use

Dose: intravenous infusion: 0.5 to 6 μg/kg/min (start at 0.5 and increase by 0.5 to 1 μg/Kg/min increments with at least 15 minutes intervals according to need

CNS: cerebral blood flow increased; dopexamine causes nausea by its action on D_2 receptors in the chemoreceptor trigger zone

CVS: stroke volume, heart rate and cardiac output increased; systolic blood pressure increased; systemic and pulmonary vascular resistance, diastolic blood pressure, LVEDP, pulmonary artery pressure reduced; coronary blood flow increased

RS: bronchodilatation

Other: mesenteric and renal vasodilation with increased blood flow, diuresis and natriuresis; hyperglycaemia, hypokalaemia; splenic platelet sequestration; 40% of dose is bound to red cells

Metabolism: rapid tissue uptake, methylation and conjugation eliminate the drug

Contra-indications: caution with MAO inhibitors

EPHEDRINE

Structure: sympathomimetic amine; α and β-agonist

Preparation: oral, tablets 15, 30, and 60 mg, elixir 15 mg/5 ml

IV clear, colourless, aqueous solution containing 30 mg ephedrine in 1 ml

Dose: IV: 3/ 6/ 9 mg increments at minimal interval of 3 to 4 minutes. Maximum of 30 mg as tachyphylaxis ensues

CNS: stimulant effect (drug of abuse)

CVS: heart rate, stroke volume, cardiac output, myocardial oxygen consumption increased; SVR, diastolic, systolic and pulmonary pressures increased; coronary blood flow increased; splanchnic and renal vasoconstriction

RS: bronchodilator; respiratory rate and tidal volume increased; irritant to mucous membranes

Other: uterine, bladder and gastrointestinal smooth muscle relaxation; bladder sphincter tone increased; gluconeogenesis, metabolic rate and oxygen consumption increased; irritant to mucous membranes

Metabolism: up to 99% eliminated in urine unchanged; the rest by oxidation, demethylation, and hydroxylation of the aromatic part plus conjugation

Contra-indications: tachyarrythmias (especially with halothane), nausea and central stimulation

ISOPRENALINE

Structure: catecholamine; β-agonist

Preparation: oral, tablets 30mg; IV: colourless, aqueous solution adjusted to a pH of 2.5 – 2.8, containing 2mg isoprenaline hydrochloride in 2 ml, with ascorbic acid and disodium edetate; requires dilution prior to use

Dose: IV infusion: 0.02 – 0.4 μg/kg/min

CNS: stimulant

CVS: heart rate, stroke volume and cardiac output increased; SA node automaticity and AV nodal conduction increased; systemic vascular resistance and diastolic blood pressure reduced; coronary blood flow increased; splanchnic and renal vasocon-striction, but flow may improve if treating low cardiac output

RS: bronchodilation

Other: uterine and gastro-intestinal smooth muscle relaxation; gluconeogenesis increased; antigen-induced histamine release is inhibited

Metabolism: extensive first pass effect if taken orally. 15 – 75% unchanged in the urine; the rest by COMT then conjugated

NOREPINEPHRINE ACID TARTRATE

Structure: catecholamine; α (and β) agonist

Preparation: clear, colourless, aqueous solution containing 0.2 mg/ml (in 2, 4, and 20 ml ampoules) or 2 mg/ml (2 ml ampoule) with sodium metabisulphite and sodium chloride. 1 mg of norepinephrine acid tartrate contains 0.5 mg norepi-nephrine base, so the preparations contain 0.1 and 1 mg norepinephrine base/ml respectively

Dose: IV infusion 0.05 to 0.2 μg/kg/min

CNS: cerebral oxygen consumption reduced

CVS: generalised peripheral vasoconstriction, systolic and diastolic blood pressure increased; a reflex fall in heart rate occurs; cardiac output may fall slightly; coronary vasodilatation causes coronary blood flow to increase; ventricular rhythm distrubances may occur

RS: mild bronchodilatation, minute volume increases

Other: hepatic, renal and splanchnic blood flow reduced; pregnant uterus contractility increased and this may compromise foetal oxygen supply; insulin secretion reduced; renin secretion increased; mydriasis; plasma water reduced by contraction of vascular space and this increases haematocrit and plasma protein concentration

Metabolism: by MAO and COMT, which in combination produce 3-methoxy-4-hydroxy mandelic acid (VMA) in the urine. 5% excreted unchanged

Contra-indications: caution with MAO inhibitors

CLONIDINE HYDROCHLORIDE

Structure: imidazoline-aniline derivative

Preparation: oral, tablets/capsules 25, 100, 250, and 300 μg

IV: clear, colourless, aqueous solution containing 150 μg in 1 ml

Dose: oral migraine/ flushing 50 to 75 μg twice daily
oral antihypertensive 50 to 600 μg three times daily
Slow IV: 150 to 300 μg for control of hypertensive crisis

Pharmacokinetics: IV dose						
onset	peak	duration	Vd	Cl	t½	
10 min	30–60 min	3–7 H	2000	3	6–23	

CNS: analgesia

CVS: transient α_1 effect causes increased systemic vascular resistance and blood pressure; α_2 agonism produces presynaptic inhibition of sympathetic norepinephrine release with reductions in SVR, blood pressure, venous return and heart rate; cardiac contractility and output are preserved; coronary blood flow increased; renal blood flow increased; rebound tachycardia and hypertension can result from sudden withdrawal

RS: no effect

Other: plasma catecholamine and renin reduced; blood glucose increased; reduction of MAC; may cause dizziness, drowsiness, headache, dry mouth and impotence

Metabolism: 65% unchanged in urine, 20% in faeces, 15% inactivated in liver

LABETALOL HYDROCHLORIDE

Structure: 2-hydroxy-5-[1-hydroxy-2-(1 methyl-3-phenyl-propylamino) ethyl] benzamide hydrochloride; combined α_1 and β_1 & β_2 adrenergic antagonist

Preparation: tablets 50, 100, 200, 400 mg; IV: clear, colourless, aqueous solution containing 100 mg in 20 ml

Dose: oral 100 to 1200 mg twice daily; IV slow bolus of 50 mg at 5 minute intervals until blood pressure is controlled (duration 6 to 18 hours, maximum dose 200 mg); IV infusion 15 – 160 mg/h

Pharmacokinetics:		
Vd	Cl	$t\frac{1}{2}$
10	23	6

CNS: fatigue, confusion

CVS: heart rate, contractility, stroke volume, cardiac output, systemic vascular resistance, systolic and diastolic blood pressure decrease; coronary and renal blood flow increased

RS: potential risk of bronchoconstriction in asthmatics

Other: with intravenous use there is a compensatory increase in endogenous catecholamines; renin and angiotensin II reduced; platelet aggregation may be reduced

Metabolism: hepatic

Contra-indications: as for other β blockers; may interact with anti-arrhythmics of Class I and IV; labetalol crosses the placenta and causes clinical effects in the foetus including bradycardia, hypotension, respiratory depression, hypoglycaemia and hypothermia in the neonate

PROPRANOLOL

Structure: 1-isopropylamino-3-(1-naphthyloxy) propan-2-ol hydrochloride

Preparation: tablets 10, 40, 80, 160 mg; IV: clear, colourless, aqueous solution containing 1 mg propranolol in 1 ml

Dose: IV: 1 to 10 mg in increments

Pharmacokinetics:		
Vd	Cl	$t\frac{1}{2}$
3.6	700	3

CNS: anxiolysis, tremor reduced, intra-ocular pressure reduced; antihypertnsive effect may have a central component

CVS: negative inotrope and chronotrope; stroke volume, heart rate, cardiac output and blood pressure reduced

RS: bronchoconstriction, airways resistance and response to hypercapnia reduced

Other: uterine tone (especially during pregnancy) reduced

Metabolism: high first pass effect and less than 1% excreted unchanged; oxidative deamination and dealkylation with subsequent glucuronidation

Contra-indications: bronchospasm in asthmatics, masks hypoglycaemia in diabetics, exacerbates peripheral vascular disease

ATROPINE SULPHATE

Structure: tertiary amine; muscarinic, anticholinergic antagonist

Preparation: oral, tablets 600 μg; IV/IM: clear, colourless, aqueous solution containing a racemic mixture of 600 μg atropine in 1 ml

Dose: 10 to 20 μg/kg

CNS: variable stimulation or depression, anti-emetic, anti Parkinsonian; competitive antagonism of muscarinic receptors cause blockade of parasympathetic system, and sweating

CVS: heart rate, AV nodal transmission and cardiac output increase (initial, temporary bradycardia with low doses due to centrally mediated increase in vagal tone); blood pressure may increase; tachyarrythmias

RS: bronchodilator with increased anatomical deadspace; respiratory rate increased; secretions reduced

Pharmacokinetics:					
Bioavailability	protein binding	pKa	Vd	Cl	t½
10–25%	50%	9.8	3	17	150

Other: gastro-intestinal motility and secretions reduced; biliary antispasmodic effect; lower oesophageal sphincter pressure reduced; urinary tract tone and peristalsis reduced, bladder sphincter tone increased and retention may result; pupillary dilatation, inabilty to accommodate for near objects (may persist for several days) and raised intra-ocular pressure occur; metabolic rate increased

Metabolism: The atropine ester is hydrolysed into its component parts tropine and tropic acid by the liver, 94% of the dose appearing in the urine in 24 hours

Contra-indications: beware glaucoma, hyperpyrexia especially in children; central anticholinergic syndrome

GLYCOPYRROLATE

Structure: quaternary amine; muscarinic anticholinergic antagonist

Preparation: IV: clear, colourless, aqueous solution containing 200 μg/ ml, 1 ml and 3 ml ampoules

Dose: IV: 4 to 5 μg/kg (10 to 15 μg/kg in conjunction with neostigmine)
Children 4 to 8 μg/kg (10 μg/kg in conjunction with neostigmine 50 μg/kg)

Pharmacokinetics:			
Bioavailability	Vd	Cl	t½
5%	0.04	0.89	50

CNS: does not cross the blood brain barrier so there is no effect on the eye; competitive antagonism of muscarinic receptors cause blockade of parasympathetic system and sweating

CVS: heart rate, AV nodal transmission and cardiac output increase, blood pressure may increase; tachyarrythmias less common than with atropine

RS: bronchodilatation with increased anatomical deadspace; secretions reduced

Other: gastro-intestinal motility and secretions reduced; lower oesophageal sphincter pressure reduced; urinary tract tone and peristalsis reduced, bladder sphincter tone increased and retention may result; metabolic rate increased

Metabolism: excreted unchanged in the urine (85%) and faeces (15%)

Contra-indications: in high doses the quaternary ammonium has a nicotinic antagonist effect of significance in myasthenia gravis; limited crossing of the placenta but can still cause foetal tachycardia

HYOSCINE HYDROBROMIDE OR BUTYLBROMIDE

Structure: tertiary amine, muscarinic anticholinergic antagonist laevo isomer used – hyoscine-1 (scopolamine)

Presentation: hyoscine-N-butylbromide; tablets 10 mg, IV: clear colourless solution, 20 mg in 1 ml: hyoscine hydrobromide 20 mg in 5 ml

Pharmacokinetics:				
Bioavailability	protein binding	Vd	Cl	t½
10%	11%	2	10	150

CNS: sedation, anti-emesis, anti Parkinsonian

CVS: initial tachycardia given IV, but may later cause bradycardia due to central effect

RS: decreases secretions, bronchodilatation, slight ventilatory stimulation

Others: antisialagogue, antispasmodic for biliary tree, and uterus; marked decrease in tear and sweat formation; decreases bladder and ureteric tone

Elimination: metabolised in the liver to scopine and scopic acid; unchanged, urine 2%, bile 5%

Toxicity: potential problem in patients with porphyria

GLYCERYL TRINITRATE

Structure: organic nitrate ester of nitric acid and glycerol (glycerine)

Preparation: sublingual tablets and oral spray, transdermal patches (5 and 10 mg), IV: clear colourless, aqueous solution containing 1 mg glyceryl trinitrate per ml with polyethylene glycol and dextrose; stored in amber ampoules with 5 and 50 ml of solution

Dose: SL: 300 μg; TD: 5 or 10 mg per 24 hours; IV: 0.2 – 3 μg/kg/min

Pharmacokinetics:		
Vd	Cl	t½
0.04 – 2.9	600	2

CNS: intracranial pressure increased as a result of vasodilatation and headache ensues if sublingual dose continues beyond desired anti-anginal effect

CVS: venodilator with arrterial dilatation as dose increases; SVR, systolic, diastolic, venous and pulmonary artery pressures reduced, myocardial oxygen demand reduced; cardiac output and coronary blood flow little effected; heart rate is unchanged in failure but increased reflexly in normal state

RS: bronchodilatation and may increase shunt

Other: relaxes other smooth muscle such as bilairy and gut

Metabolism: hydrolysis of the ester bonds by red cells and the liver, and 80% of the dose is excreted in the urine

Contra-indications: substantial amount of intravenously administered GTN binds to the plastic of giving sets and syringes, therefore reduced availability

SODIUM NITROPRUSSIDE

Structure: inorganic complex

Preparation: red-brown powder containing 50 mg sodium nitroprusside in a brown glass ampoule which is reconstituted in 2 ml 5% dextrose prior to further dilution. It should be protected from light and yellow and brown giving sets and syringes are available for this purpose.

Dose: IV infusion 0.1 – 1.5 μg/kg/min (maximum of up to 8 μg/kg/min)

Maximum dose 1.5 mg/kg; starts to accumulates once rate exceeds 2 μg/kg/min

Pharmacokinetics:

Vd	Elimination	nitroprusside t½	thiocyanate t½
200	1 μg/kg/min	very short	2.7 days

CNS: cerebral vasodilatation increases intracranial pressure

CVS: dilates arterioles and venules with reduced blood pressure, reduced LVEDP, reduced myocardial oxygen demand; heart rate increases but contractility is unaffected.

RS: hypoxic pulmonary vasoconstriction is impaired and arterial oxygen tension may fall

Other: gastro-intestinal motility and lower oesophageal sphincter pressure are reduced; metabolic acidosis may occur

Metabolism: reacts with sulphydryl groups of plasma amino acids; higher concentrations cause non-enzymatic hydrolysis in red blood cells to produce five cyanide ions from each nitroprusside molecule. One of these combines with haemoglobin (iron in ferrous state) to form methaemoglobin (iron in ferric state); most of the rest is converted to thiocyanate by rhodonase in the liver and is then excreted in the urine; small amount of thiocyanate combines with vitamin B_{12} to form cyanocobalamin

Toxicity: cyanide ions inhibit the cytochrome oxidase chain; plasma levels of above 80 μg/l produce tachycardia, sweating, hyperventilation, cardiac arrrhythmias and retrosternal pain

CARDIOVASCULAR PHARMACOLOGY

terminal half life (t½) – hours unless otherwise stated

ADENOSINE

Structure: a nucleoside comprising adenine (6-amino purine) and D-ribofuranose (pentose sugar)

Presentation: IV: clear, aqueous solution of adenosine 6 mg in 2 ml of 0.9% sodium chloride

Dose: IV: bolus 3 mg over 2 seconds, then bolus 6 mg after 1–2 minutes if necessary, then bolus 12 mg after 1–2 minutes if necessary; stop if high nodal block develops

Pharmacokinetics: t½ 8–10 s

CNS: rare occurrence of blurred vision, headache, dizziness

CVS: inhibits AV nodal conduction, reduces contractility, vasodilatation; palpitations, flushing, hypotension, severe bradycardia may occur

RS: dyspnoea, bronchospasm may occur

Other effects: nausea

Elimination: rapid cellular uptake, adenosine deaminase, phosphorylation to nucleotide

Contra-indications: second and third degree heart block and sick sinus syndrome unless artificial pacemaker functioning; asthma

Interactions: dipyridamole inhibits adenosine uptake (if essential use 0.5 – 1 mg dose); xanthines (caffeine, aminophylline) are potent inhibitors of adenosine; drugs slowing AV nodal conduction

AMIODARONE HYDROCHLORIDE

Structure: iodinated benzofuran derivative – class III anti-arrhythmic

Presentation: tablets 200 mg, 100 mg; IV: clear, pale yellow solution 150mg in 3ml

Dose: oral loading regimen then 200 mg/day; IV 5mg/kg over 20 min to 2 hours onset of action by oral route is 6 days

Pharmacokinetics:		
bioavailability	protein binding	t½
22–86%	97%	1300

CNS: peripheral neuropathy rare; nightmares, tremor, ataxia; corneal microdeposits (benign and reversible

CVS: slows heart rate and may cause bradycardia, and AV block

RS: may rarely cause diffuse pulmonary alveolitis and fibrosis

Other effects: metabolite blocks conversion of T3 to thyroxine and may therefore cause hypo- or hyper-thyroidism. thyroid function should be monitored. It may cause chronic liver disease, and transaminases often rise, especially at start of treatment

Elimination: it is deiodinated and has a very long half-life because it is highly lipid soluble and highly tissue bound which may result in cumulation; toxic effects may still be present months after treatment stopped

DIGOXIN

Structure: sterol lactone with sugar moiety – cardiac glycoside

Presentation: tablets 62.5, 125 and 250 μg, elixir. IV: clear, colourless, aqueous solution, 125 μg/ml

Dose: IV: up to 1 mg loading dose by slow (25 μg/min) injection; typically 10 μg/kg once daily oral or IV, monitor levels, plasma concentrations (nmol/l): therapeutic 1.3–1.5; toxic 3.5

Pharmacokinetics:

bioavailability	protein binding	Vd	t½
75%	25%	8	35

Clearance $= 0.88 \times$ creatinine clearance $+ 0.33$

CNS: nausea, vomiting, dizziness, anorexia, fatigue, apathy, malaise, visual disturbance, depression and psychosis

CVS: positive inotropy, especially in hypervolaemic failure; negative chronotropy; slowing of AV conduction; in excess may cause complete heart block, and most rhythm disturbances especially bradycardias

Other effects: mild intrinsic diuretic affect; abdominal pain, diarrhoea; gynaecomastia (steroid related); intestinal necrosis (oral route); skin rashes; thrombocytopoenia

Elimination: 10% metabolised in the liver by progressive removal of the sugar moieties; 60% excreted unchanged in the urine by glomerular filtration and active tubular secretion. Toxicity increased by low potassium, low magnesium, high sodium, high calcium, acid-base disturbance and hypoxaemia. Poorly removed by dialysis as highly tissue bound; digoxin specific antibody fragments available for treatment of poisoning.

DILTIAZEM

Structure: benzothiapine calcium antagonist – class IV anti-arrhythmic

Presentation: tablets 60mg

Dose: 60 – 120 mg, 6–8 hourly

Pharmacokinetics:

bioavailability	protein binding	Vd	Cl	t½
35%	80%	5.3	15	5

CNS: no effect

CVS: causes peripheral and coronary arterial vasodilatation; decreases systemic and peripheral resistance; slows AV nodal conduction; exacerbates the negative inotropic effects of volatile agents

RS: antihistamine effect

Other effects: renal artery dilatation increases renal plasma flow local anaesthetic effect; reduced lower oesophageal sphincter pressure in achalasia; may inhibit platelet aggregation

Elimination: 2% is excreted unchanged in the urine; de-acetylation and demethylation produce active metabolites which are conjugated with glucuronides and sulphates; renal failure has no effect on elimination

ESMOLOL HYDROCHLORIDE

Structure: aryloxypropanolamine – β blocker – class II anti-arrhythmic

Presentation: IV: clear, aqueous solution 10 ml of 250 mg/ml for dilution and infusion; 10 ml of 100 mg/ml for undiluted boluses

Dose: 50–200 μg/kg/min; a loading dose may be used

Pharmacokinetics:			
protein binding	Vd	Cl	t½
56%	3.43	285	9.2 minutes

CVS: mainly β_1; used for acute SVT, acute control of hypertension and myocardial infarction; negative chronotrope and inotrope, cardiac output falls by 20%

RS: selectivity minimises increases in airway resistance

Elimination: metabolised by red cell esterases producing methanol and a primary acid (70–80% as this in urine) that has weak β antagonism and half life of 3.5 hours; less than 1% is excreted unchanged in the urine. Use with caution in renal failure; hepatic failure has no effect

NIFEDIPINE

Structure: dihydropyridine calcium antagonist- class IV antidysrrhythmic

Presentation: tablets 10 & 20 mg and capsules 5 & 10 mg; the yellow, viscous liquid in the capsules has been used sublingually for speedy control of blood pressure; a solution is available for direct intra-coronary injection

Dose: oral 10–20 mg 8 hourly, 20–40 mg 12 hourly slow release formulation

Pharmacokinetics:				
bioavailability	protein binding	Vd	Cl	t½
65%	95%	0.8	10	5

CNS: marginal increase in cerebral blood flow; headache, flushing, dizziness

CVS: decreases systemic and peripheral vascular resistance, decreases pulmonary artery pressure, reflex increase in heart rate and cardiac output; increases epicardial and coronary blood flow, negative inotrope

RS: no effect

Other effects: increases red cell deformability, decreases platelet aggregation, decreases thromboxane synthesis; reduces lower oesophageal sphincter pressure; increases renin, increases catecholamines; increases hepatic blood flow; oedema of legs; eye pain; gum hyperplasia

Elimination: 85% in urine; 15% in bile; non cumulative

VERAPAMIL

Structure: synthetic papaverine derivative – class IV antiarrhythmic

Presentation: tablets 40, 80 and 120 mg. IV: 5 mg in 2 ml (racemic mixture of l and d isomers)

Dose: oral 40–120 mg 8 hourly; IV 10 mg (0.075–0.20 mg/kg)

Pharmacokinetics:			
bioavailability	protein binding	Vd	t½
20%	90%	4.5	5

CNS: dizziness, headache

CVS: slows cardiac action potential; slows AV nodal conduction; decreases systemic vascular resistance; decreases blood pressure heart rate and cadiac output; increases coronary blood flow

RS: no effect

Other effects: local anaesthetic effect; constipation

Elimination: 70% excreted in urine as conjugated metabolites, 5% unchanged; non-cumulative;

half life is increased in hepatic disease

Interactions: avoid concurrent use with β blocker as it may cause asystole or hypotension

RESPIRATORY PHARMACOLOGY

AMINOPHYLLINE

Structure: ethylene diamine salt of the methylxanthine theophylline

Presentation: tablets 100 mg; IV clear solution 25 mg/ml; sustained release preparations also available

Dose: oral up to 300 mg three times daily; IV cautious slow infusion 500 μg/kg/H adjusted by serum theophylline concentrations

CNS: direct respiratory stimulant, may cause convulsions

CVS: myocardial contractility and heart rate rise, cardiac output increased; marked peripheral vasodilatation (offset slightly by vasomotor centre stimulation)

RS: bronchodilatation by β_2 action, direct respiratory centre stimulation; rise in respiratory rate

Other: general smooth muscle relaxation; renal blood flow increased

Elimination: demethylation and oxidation in the liver followed by urinary excretion

Caution: rapid IV administration my result in convulsions, tachycardia and collapse

BECLAMETHASONE

Structure: synthetic corticosteroid

Presentation: metered inhaler, 50 100 or 200 μg per puff

Dose: up to maximum of 800 μg daily (adult)

CNS: steroid psychosis rare but possible in high dosage

CVS: hypertension and fluid retention possible in high dosage

RS: reduction in airway sensitivity, reduction of bronchospasm; risk of candida albicans infection

Other: adrenal suppression possible; ostetoporosis is a risk in chronic therapy

BUDESONIDE

Structure: synthetic corticosteroid

Presentation: metered inhaler, 50 or 200 μg per puff

Dose: 200–400 μg twice daily

CNS: steroid psychosis rare but possible in high dosage

CVS: hypertension and fluid retention possible in high dosage

RS: reduction in airway sensitivity, reduction of bronchospasm; risk of candida albicans infection

Other: adrenal suppression possible; osteoporosis a risk in chronic therapy

CROMOGLYCATE DISODIUM

Structure: organic cogener of khellin

Presentation: metered inhaler, 5 mg per puff, spincap® 20 mg, nebuliser solution 10 mg/ml (also available as eye drops)

Dose: up to 20 mg four times daily; duration of single dose 6 H

Pharmacokinetics:		
Bioavailability	protein binding	t½
10%	70%	90

CNS: no effect

CVS: no effect

RS: prophylactic against brochospasm; may produce coughing and throat irritation

Other: used in food allergy and inflammatory eye conditions

DOXAPRAM

Structure: monohydrated pyrrolidinone

Presentation: IV clear, colourless solution 100mg in 5ml, or 2mg/ml in 500 ml of 5% dextrose

Dose: IV: 1 to 1.5 mg/kg onset 30 s, peak 2 m, lasts 10 min

Pharmacokinetics:		
Vd	Cl	$t\frac{1}{2}$
1.5	5	3 H

CNS: carotid body chemoreceptors and repiratory centre stimulation; higher doses cause restlessness, dizziness, headache, hallucinations, convulsions

CVS: stroke volume and cardiac output increased; heart rate and blood pressure may increase

RS: tidal volume increased; rate increased with higher doses or if slow; minute volume increased. carbon dioxide response curve shifted to left

Other: may increase urine output, salivation, and motility of GI and urinary tracts

Elimination: 95% metabolised primarily by liver, 5% unchanged in urine

Side-effects: potentiates sympathomimetic amines; increased effect if on MAOI; may cause agitation and increased skeletal muscle activity when concurrent with aminophylline therapy

Caution: if respiratory failure not due to inadequate respiratory drive, will cause agitation and convulsions

IPATROPIUM BROMIDE

Structure: quaternary derivative of N-isopropyl atropine

Presentation: Aerocap® 40 mg dry powder formulation, metered inhaler 20 µg per puff, nebuliser solution 250 µg/ml also available; maximum effect 30 min after administration, duration 6 h

Dose: up to 40 µg three times daily

CNS: no effect

CVS: no effect

RS: brochodilatation, occasional irritation and cough; paradoxical bronchospasm possible but rare

Other: may produce glaucoma and urinary retention (anticholinergic effects)

SALBUTAMOL

Structure: synthetic amine

Presentation: IV clear solution 5 mg in 5 ml, tablets 4 and 8 mg, syrup 2 mg in 5 ml, inhalation powder 200 and 400 µg, nebuliser solution 5 mg/ml

Dose: IV 250 µg bolus; 3 to 20 µg/min by infusion

Pharmacokinetics:			
protein binding	Vd	Cl	t½
8 to 64%	2.2	6.7	4 H

CNS: may cause excitation, anxiety, tremor

CVS: β_2 effects cause vasodilatation with decreased blood pressure; higher doses cause β_1 effects with tachycardia

RS: bronchodilator for prophylactic and therapeutic use

Other: crosses placenta and may causes foetal tachycardia

Elimination: 30% unchanged in urine; the rest unchanged in faeces, small amount of conjugated form also appears in urine and faeces

ENDOCRINE PHARMACOLOGY

HYDROCORTISONE

Structure: glucocorticoid steroid

Presentation: IV/IM, white powder as sodium succinate for reconstitution with water for injection (many other preparations are available)

Dose: IV 100–500 mg 6 to 8 hourly, onset 2–4 H, lasts 8 H

CNS: mood changes

CVS: restores vasomotor tone of small blood vessels, reduces vascular permeability and resultant tissue swelling

RS: reduces bronchial wall swelling caused by asthma or anaphylaxis

Other: anti-inflammatory agent with multiple uses

Elimination: hepatic conversion to tetrahydrocrtisone

Side-effects: anaphylactoid reactions have occurred

Cautions: congestive cardiac failure, hypertension, peptic ulceration, glaucoma, epilepsy, diabetes mellitus, history of tuberculosis, effect of anticholinesterases antagonised

DEXAMETHASONE

Structure: glucocorticoid steroid

Presentation: IV, clear, colourless solution; 8 mg dexamethasone in 2 ml

Dose: IV: 0.5 to 20 mg initial bolus, particularly indicated where sodium and water retention are to be avoided

CNS: may cause convulsions and increase ICP (but indicated for treatment of cerebral oedema)

CVS: minimal effect

RS: may be used for asthma and aspiration pneumonitis

Other: mineralocorticoid effects may be present to a limited extent

Elimination: liver metabolised

Side-effects: as for hydrocortisone

INSULIN (SOLUBLE)

Structure: glycopeptide; formed as pro-insulin with a connecting peptide, the C fragment

Presentation: clear colourless solution of human insulin pH 6.6–8.0 (containing glycerol and m-cresol)

Dose: SC/IM/IV, typically up to 8 IU/H based on intermittent blood glucose monitoring; used as replacement for low endogenous insulin, may be necessary in total parenteral nutrition to facilitate glucose absorption

OXYTOCIN

Structure: synthetic octapeptide identical to human oxytocin

Presentation: IV/IM, clear, colourless solution, 5 or 10 IU in 1ml (available in combination with ergometrine 500 μg in 1 ml, as syntometrine)

Dose: IV to augment labour by infusion of variable magnitude; following Caesarean delivery slow bolus of 5 or 10 IU

CNS: no effect

CVS: bolus administration causes transient hypotension with reflex tachycardia. Following term delivery usually offset by placental autotransfusion

RS: no effect

Others: breast duct smooth muscle contraction promoting milk ejection

Elimination: rapid metabolism by plasma oxytocinase (use separate line if transfusing blood or plasma)

Side-effects: uterine spasm or rupture, hypotension, water intoxication (secondary to the ADH like effect)

ERGOMETRINE MALEATE

Structure: ergot alkaloid

Presentation: IV/IM, colourless solution, 500 μg in 1 ml (available in combination with oxytocin, see above)

Dose: slow IV 125 – 250 μg; IM 500 μg

CNS: potent emetic, avoid in pre-eclampsia

CVS: direct vasoconstriction, avoid in hypertension

RS: occasional dyspnoea, chest tightness

Side-effects: nausea, vomiting, vasoconstriction (potential for stroke, myocardial infaction)

Contraindications: induction of labour, first and second stages of labour; avoid in prescence of cardiac or vascular disease, or porphyria

GASTRO-INTESTINAL PHARMACOLOGY

CARBENOXOLONE

Structure: derivative of glycyrrhizic acid

Presentation: tablets 20 mg, liquid 10 mg, combined with aluminium hydroxide

Dose: 20 mg three times daily after meals

CNS: confusion and coma possible if water retention severe

CVS: risk of hypertension and failure secondary to sodium and water retention

RS: no effect

Other effects: muscle weakness; hypokalaemia

Contra-indications: cardiac failure, hypokalaemia, heptaic and renal impairment

CIMETIDINE

Structure: histamine related imidazole ring

Presentation: tablets 200 mg, 400 mg, 800 mg, suspension 100 mg in 5 ml

Dose: 400 mg twice daily

CNS: headache, dizziness, confusion

CVS: bradycardia, AV block, hypotension

Pharmacokinetics:

Bioavailability	protein binding	Vd	t½
60%	20%	1–2	1–2.5 H

RS: no effect

Other effects: gynaecomastia; impotence; thrombocytopaenia; muscle pains ; occasionally pancreatitis

OMEPRAZOLE

Structure: substituted benzimidazole

Presentation: tablets 10 mg, 20 mg, 40 mg

Dose: 20 mg daily, increasing to 40 mg daily

Pharmacokinetics:

Bioavailability	protein binding	peak plasma levels	t½	pKa
35%	95%	20 min	60	3.97

CNS: headache, dizziness

CVS: no effect

RS: no effect

Other effects: rash; pruritus; eosinophilia; gynaecomastia; liver dysfunction

RANITIDINE

Structure: furan derivative – 5-membered oxygen containing ring with three tertiary amine groups in the side chains

Presentation: tablets 150mg and 300mg; clear aqueous solution (50mg in 2ml) for IV/IM use

Dose: slow intravenous bolus 50mg 6–8 hourly; oral 150mg twice daily

Pharmacokinetics:

Bioavailability	protein binding	Vd	Cl	t½
50–60%	15%	1.5	10	120

CNS: no effect

CVS: no effect

RS: no effect

Other effects: placenta is readily crossed

Interactions: the increase in gastric pH increases the non-ionised proportion of some drugs (such as benzodiazepines) and so increases their absorption

ANTICOAGULANTS

Anticoagulants are drugs that interfere with the process of fibrin plug formation to reduce or prevent coagulation. This effect is used to reduce the risk of thrombus formation within normal vessels and vascular grafts. The injectable anticoagulants are also used to prevent coagulation in extracorporeal circuits and in blood product storage. There are two main types of anticoagulants: the oral anticoagulants and the injectable anticoagulants (heparins).

ORAL ANTICOAGULANTS

Oral anticoagulants inhibit the reduction of vitamin K. Reduced vitamin K is required as a cofactor in γ-carboxylation of the glutamate residues of the glycoprotein clotting factors II, VII, IX and X, which are synthesised in the liver. During this γ-carboxylation process, vitamin K is oxidised to vitamin K-2,3-epoxide. The oral anticoagulants prevent the reduction of this compound back to vitamin K. In order to work, coumarins must be utilised in the liver. The oral anticoagulants do this by virtue of their structural similarity to vitamin K. Their action depends on the depletion of these factors, which decline according to their individual half-lives (see below).

HALF-LIVES OF VITAMIN K-DEPENDENT CLOTTING FACTORS	
Factor	Half life (H)
II	60
VII	6
IX	24
X	40

There are two groups of oral anticoagulants:

- coumarins (warfarin and nicoumalone)
- inandiones (phenindione)

Warfarin has the most widespread use. Phenindione is more likely to cause hypersensitivity, but is useful when there is intolerance to warfarin.

Warfarin sodium

Warfarin is administered orally as a racemic mixture of D and L warfarin. It is rapidly absorbed reaching a peak plasma concentration within an hour with a bio-availability of 100%. However, a clinical effect is not apparent until the clotting factors become depleted after 12 to 16 hours and reaching a peak at 36 to 48 hours. Warfarin is 99% protein bound (to albumin) in the plasma resulting in a small volume of distribution. Warfarin is metabolised in the liver by oxidation (*L*-form) and reduction (*D*-form), followed by glucuronide conjugation, with a half-life of about 40 hours.

Warfarin crosses the placenta and is teratogenic during pregnancy, and postpartum it passes into the milk. This is a particular problem as the gut flora responsible for producing vitamin K_2 and hepatic function in the newborn are not fully developed.

Warfarin has a low therapeutic index and is particularly prone to interactions with other drugs. Interactions increasing the effect of warfarin occur in several ways:

- competition for protein binding sites
- increased hepatic binding
- inhibition of hepatic microsomal enzymes
- reduced vitamin K synthesis
- synergistic anti-haemostatic actions

Drugs such as NSAID's, chloral hydrate, oral hypoglycaemic agents, diuretics and amiodarone displace warfarin from albumin binding sites resulting in higher free plasma levels and greater effect. This effect is made more significant because normally only 1% of warfarin is free and a small change in protein binding has a dramatic effect on free warfarin levels. *D*-thyroxine increases the potency of warfarin by increasing hepatic binding. Ethanol ingestion may inhibit liver enzymes responsible for warfarin elimination. The effect of warfarin may also be increased by acute illness, low vitamin K intake and drugs such as cimetidine, aminoglycosides and paracetamol. Broad-spectrum antibiotics reduce the level of gut bacteria responsible for vitamin K_2 synthesis, and may enhance the effect of warfarin where the diet is deficient in vitamin K. Other anticoagulants and particularly anti-platelet drugs increase the clinical effects of warfarin.

Interactions decreasing the effect of warfarin can occur in several ways, notably:

- induction of hepatic microsomal enzymes
- drugs that increase levels of clotting factors
- binding of warfarin
- increased vitamin K intake

The effect of warfarin may be reduced by induction of hepatic enzymes by barbiturates and phenytoin. Oestrogens increase the production of vitamin-K dependent clotting factors (II, VII, IX, X). Cholestyramine binds warfarin reducing its effect. Carbamazepine and rifampicin reduce the effect of warfarin but the mechanism of this effect is not clear.

HEPARINS

Heparins are injectable anticoagulants that act by binding to antithrombin resulting in a profound increase in antithrombin activity.

Structure
Heparin is a group of sulphated acid glycosaminoglycans (or mucopolysaccharides) comprising alternate monosaccharide residues of N-acetylglucosamine and

glucuronic acid and their derivatives. The glucuronic acid residues are mostly in the iduronic acid form and some are ester-sulphated. The N-acetylglucosamine residues may be deacylated, N-sulphated and ester-sulphated in a random manner. This results in a chain of 45 to 50 sugar residues of variable composition based on the above units. The molecules are attached by the sulphated components to a protein skeleton consisting entirely of glycine and serine amino acid residues. The molecular weight of heparin ranges from 3000 to 40000, with a mean of 12000 to 15000. Endogenous heparin is located in the lungs, in arterial walls and in mast cells as large polymers of molecular weight 750 000. It is present in the plasma at a concentration of 1.5 mg/l.

Heparin has a strong negative charge and is a large molecule, so there is minimal absorption following oral administration. It supplied as heparin sodium and heparin calcium.

Mechanism of action
Heparin has the following effects:

- inhibition of coagulation by enhancing the action of antithrombin on the serine protease coagulation factors (IIa, Xa, XIIa, XIa, and IXa)
- reduced platelet aggregation
- increased vascular permeability
- release of lipoprotein lipases into plasma

The negatively charged heparin binds to the negatively charged lysine residue in antithrombin, an α_2-globulin, which in turns increases the affinity of the arginine site of antithrombin for the serine site of thrombin (Factor II). This increases the inhibitory activity of antithrombin 2300-fold. This reversible bond is the feature of a specific antithrombin binding site comprising five particular residues. This particular pentasaccharide sequence is present randomly in about a third of the heparin molecules. For full activity of heparin on thrombin (IIa) a heparin molecule must have at least 13 extra sugar residues in addition to the pentasaccharide antithrombin binding site sequence. The covalently bonded thrombin-antithrombin complex is inactive but once it is formed formed the heparin is released and the complex is rapidly destroyed by the liver. The active heparin section is then free to act on more antithrombin. Heparin acts in a similar way on the other activated serine protease coagulation factors (XIIa, XIa, and IXa). The binding of heparin to both the clotting factor and antithrombin is important in the above enhancement of antithrombin. The activity of heparin on factor Xa is also mediated by increasing the affinity of antithrombin for the clotting factor but heparin does not bind to factor Xa. Factor Xa inhibition is enhanced with lower levels of heparin than those required for thrombin inhibition. Heparin reduces platelet aggregation secondary to the reduction in thrombin (a potent platelet aggregator). The increase in plasma lipase results in an increase in free fatty acid levels.

Low molecular weight heparins

Examples: certoparin, enoxaparin, tinzaparin)

The low molecular weight (LMW) heparins are fragments of depolymerised heparin purified to contain the antithrombin specific binding site. Therefore, they all inhibit factor Xa. The molecular weight of LMW heparins ranges from 3000 to 8000 Daltons, with a mean of 4000 to 6500. They comprise 13 to 22 sugar residues. The LMW heparins have a full anti-Xa activity but much reduced antithrombin activity and require the prescence of antithrombin for their effect. The reduction in interference with thrombin gives LMW heparins the following advantages:

- minimal alteration of platelet function
- better intra-operative haemostasis
- possible better venous thromboembolic prophylaxis in orthopaedic practice

Administration
Heparin is administered intravenously and subcutaneously. A typical adult dose for thrombosis prophylaxis is 5000 IU subcutaneously 8 to 12 hourly. For full anticoagulation, as used during cardiopulmonary bypass, a dose of 3 mg/kg (300 IU/kg) is used to achieve 3 to 4 IU heparin/ml of blood. Heparin has an immediate action within the plasma. Heparin has a volume of distribution of 40 to 100 ml/kg and is bound to antithrombin, albumin, fibrinogen and proteases. Increase in acute phase proteins (during acute illness) can significantly alter the clinical effect. Heparin also binds to platelet and endothelial protein, reducing bioavailability and effect. The drug is metabolised in the liver, kidney and reticulo-endothelial system by heparinases that desulphate the mucopolysaccharide residues and hydrolyse the links between them. Heparin has a half-life of 40 to 90 minutes.

Low molecular weight heparins are also administered subcutaneously and have the advantage of once daily administration. They may be used in extracorporeal dialysis circuits, and have been used in cardiopulmonary bypass. LMW heparins are much less bound to proteins in the plasma, platelets and vascular walls and bioavailability after subcutaneous administration is at least 90%. The levels of free LMW heparin are therefore much more predictable and require less monitoring. Peak anti-Xa activity is achieved within 3 to 4 hours after subcutaneous injection and activity has halved after 12 hours. Elimination is predominantly renal and half-life may be raised in renal failure.

Effects on coagulation studies
Heparin increases APTT, TT, ACT but does not affect bleeding time. Heparin therapy is routinely checked using the APTT, and, on cardiopulmonary bypass, using ACT.

Heparin relies on the presence of antithrombin for its activity. Prolonged heparin therapy may lead to osteoporosis by an unknown mechanism.

Protamine
Protamine is a group of basic, cationic (positively charged) proteins of relatively low molecular weight. Protamine is used to neutralise the effects of heparin and LMW heparins. This occurs because the negative charge of the heparin is attracted to the positive charges of the protamine. 1 mg of protamine sulphate neutralises 1 mg (100 IU) of heparin. Protamine itself (in excess), has anticoagulant activity although this is effect is not as powerful as that of heparin.

CALCIUM CHELATING AGENTS

Calcium is an essential cofactor in the coagulation system. Agents that bind calcium will therefore inhibit coagulation. Citrate is used to bind calcium in stored blood to prevent its coagulation. In vivo, the citrate is metabolised by the liver reversing this inhibition. However, massive transfusion may temporarily overload the liver's capacity to metabolise citrate particularly if metabolic rate is reduced by cooling by the transfusion itself or by deliberate cooling as used in cardiac surgery. To some extent this may be overcome by administering calcium ions.

FIBRINOLYTIC AGENTS

Fibrinolysis may be **activated** or **inhibited** pharmacologically.

PLASMINOGEN ACTIVATORS

Examples: alteplase, reteplase, streptokinase, urokinase

The plasminogen activators act by catalysing the conversion of plasminogen to plasmin, the enzyme responsible for the enzymatic degradation of fibrin clot. Plasminogen activators are used to destroy clots in the following situations:

- venous thrombosis
- pulmonary embolus
- retinal thrombosis
- myocardial infarction

The drugs may also remove clot formed in response to haemorrhage, so bleeding from other sites is a risk. In some cases this can be minimised by administering the activator directly to the desired site of thrombus by catheter. However, this is technically difficult and the delay in doing so may remove any benefit. Some of these agents require heparin and or aspirin to prevent reformation of thrombus. They may reduce levels of plasminogen, α_2-antiplasmin, α_2-macroglobulin and C_1-esterase inhibitor.

Alteplase (rt-PA) is a synthetic form of tissue-type plasminogen activator (a glycoprotein). Anistreplase is a ready combined complex of plasminogen and streptokinase that is blocked by an anisoyl group. Once in the body the anisoyl group leaves the complex, which produces plasmin and so activates fibrinolysis. Reteplase is another recombinant plasminogen activator. These three agents act on fibrin-bound plasminogen. Streptokinase is obtained from group C *haemolytic Streptococci* cultures. Streptokinase induces an immune response that produces antibodies to the drug and limits its useful duration to 6 days. Allergy is common. Patients frequently have antibodies to protein from previous exposure to the Streptococcus. Urokinase is derived from human kidney cell cultures or urine and is therefore non-antigenic.

FIBRINOLYTIC INHIBITORS

Examples: aprotinin, tranexamic acid

The fibrinolytic inhibitors act by inhibiting the enzymatic activity of plasmin on fibrin. They are used to prevent the breakdown of fibrin clot when excessive bleeding during surgery is a risk. Uses include the reduction of blood loss during surgery in haemophiliacs, cardiac surgery and in thrombolytic overdose.

Aprotinin is a polypeptide and inhibitor of proteolytic enzymes in general, but specifically used for its action on plasmin and kallikrein. It has also been tried in the treatment of acute pancreatitis. Tranexamic acid inhibits the fibrinolytic activity of both plasmin and pepsin. It is useful in upper gastro-intestinal haemorrhage and in surgery in haemophiliacs and it can be administered orally or intravenously.

ANTIPLATELET DRUGS

ASPIRIN

Aspirin irreversibly inactivates platelet cyclo-oxygenase (COX_2) by acetylation of the terminal serine amino acid. This inhibits endoperoxide and so thromboxane (TXA_2) production within the platelets. More importantly, endothelial cells generate new cyclo-oxygenase, whereas platelets are unable to. As it is an irreversible process, the effect on an individual platelet is permanent for the 4 to 6 day life span of the platelet. Aspirin is not specific for platelet cyclo-oxygenase but this is more readily inactivated than endothelial cyclo-oxygenase responsible for prostacyclin production. Aspirin should be stopped 7 to 10 days before surgery to allow regeneration of normally functioning platelets. It may be restarted 6 hours post-operatively. Prolonged aspirin usage may reduce circulating levels of factors II, VII, IX and X.

Other NSAID's also inhibit COX, but are generally less potent and the inhibition is reversible so that the overall effect on platelet function is small.

PROSTACYCLIN

Synthetic prostacyclin (epoprostenol) inhibits platelet aggregation and dissipates platelet aggregates. It can be used in haemodialysis, but must be given as an infusion as its half-life is about 3 minutes. Prostacyclin is also a potent vasodilator, so patients should be observed for hypotension, flushing and headaches.

INDEX